I0791313

ISBN: 9781670364395

MAXIMUM WEIGHT LOSS

1500 Calorie

Diet and Exercise

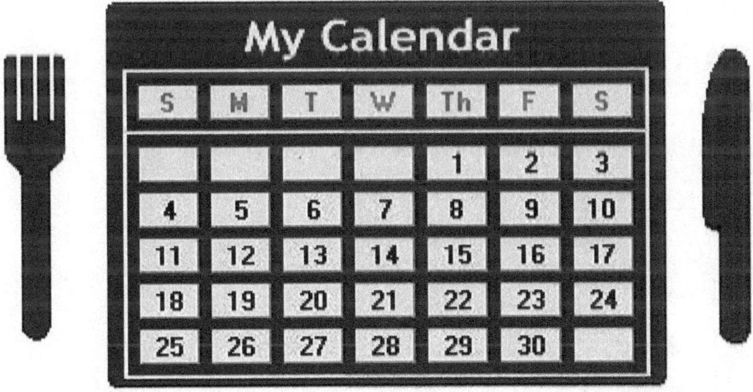

Vincent Antonetti, PhD

NoPaperPress™

Note: At publication, the off-the-shelf foods used in this book were widely available in most supermarkets. But food products come and go. So if there is a frozen entrée or soup selection in this diet that is out of stock, or that's been discontinued, or perhaps you don't like, or that you forgot to pick up while shopping, please substitute another food that has **approximately** the same caloric value and nutritional content. In this regard, many dieters have found the foods listed in the Appendices at the end of this book to be very helpful.

CONTENTS

By our lifestyle and actions, we have some control over the quality of our life. There are steps we can take to maintain our mental and physical capacity, measures that will allow us to live life to the fullest – and the longest. What is the secret? Most researchers agree that, in addition to doing something that is mentally stimulating and emotionally rewarding, a sensible regular exercise program, a nutritious diet and a healthy body weight are key.

Max Weight Loss: Why Diet & Exercise

If you want to lose some weight, choose a weight loss regimen that includes both dieting and exercise. Why? The diet reduces your calorie intake. And a good workout burns calories and builds muscle which speeds up your metabolism. Together they result in **maximum weight loss**.

What Should You Weigh

A convenient way to determine what you should weigh is to use my new BMI-Based Weight vs. Height Chart shown as Table 1, Normal weight is for BMI = 18.6 to 24.9, Overweight is for BMI = 25.0 to 29.9, and Obese is for BMI = 30.0 to 39.9.

Height	Normal	Overweight	Obese
4' 10"	90 – 119	120 – 142	143 – 191
4' 11"	93 – 123	124 – 148	149 – 197
5' 0"	96 – 127	128 – 152	153 – 204
5' 1"	99 – 131	132 – 158	159 – 211
5' 2"	102 – 135	136 – 163	164 – 218
5' 3"	105 – 140	141 – 169	170 – 225
5' 4"	109 – 144	145 – 173	174 – 232
5' 5"	112 – 149	150 – 180	181 – 239
5' 6"	116 – 154	155 – 185	186 – 247
5' 7"	119 – 159	160 – 191	192 – 254
5' 8"	123 – 163	164 – 196	197 – 262
5' 9"	126 – 168	169 – 202	203 – 270
5' 10"	130 – 173	174 – 206	207 – 278
5' 11"	134 – 178	179 – 214	215 – 286
6' 0"	137 – 183	184 – 220	221 – 294
6' 1"	141 – 188	189 – 227	228 – 302
6' 2"	145 – 194	195 – 232	233 – 310
6' 3"	149 – 199	200 – 239	240 – 319
6' 4"	152 – 205	206 - 246	247 - 328
6' 5"	157 - 210	211 - 252	253 – 337
6' 6"	161 - 216	217 - 259	260 - 346

Table 1: Weight vs. Height

Weight Loss Prediction Tables

Weight loss occurs when your food energy intake is less than the total energy you expend. This difference in calories is referred to as your <u>calorie deficit</u>. How much weight you lose depends on the magnitude of your calorie deficit. Physiologists have long known that to lose one pound requires a deficit of approximately 3,500 Calories. Therefore, if a person's total calorie deficit over time is known, their weight loss over time can be calculated. Fortunately, a more precise determination of the rate of weight loss is possible. Scientists have demonstrated that **weight loss is a function of age, sex, height, weight, physical activity, caloric intake and the duration of the diet (or time on the diet)**. This writer related all these variables in a complex, scientifically based, energy-weight-control equation, published in the *American Journal of Clinical Nutrition,*, and subsequently published a set of 60 Weight Loss Prediction tables in hardcover book *The Computer Diet*. In this edition of *Maximum Weight Loss* you will find an abridged set of six Weight Loss Prediction tables for moderately active men and women (see Table 2).

Selecting the Correct Table

Your first task is to choose the correct Weight Loss Prediction Table. The six Weight Loss Prediction Tables are organized by gender and age. Given the Workout recommended in this book, the activity level is restricted to what is called Moderate in this text: **Moderately Active**: To qualify for this category, you have to engage in some form of regular exercise <u>at least six days per week</u> (e.g., taking a brisk walk, and/or working out with weights). Use Table 2 to find the Weight Loss Prediction Table that is applicable to you.

Gender	Age	Activity Level	Table - Page
Men	18 - 35	Moderate	**3 - 9**
	36 - 55	Moderate	**4 - 10**
	56 - 75	Moderate	**5 - 11**
Women	18 - 35	Moderate	**6 - 12**
	36 - 55	Moderate	**7 - 13**
	56 - 75	Moderate	**8 - 14**

Table 2: Weight Loss Prediction Tables

WEIGHT LOSS PREDICTION FOR MEN Ages 18-35
(Moderately Active During or After Working Hours)

Weight (lbs.)	Diet Calorie	Weight Loss Desired (lbs.)							
		10	20	30	40	50	60	70	80
140	1500	34							
160.	1500	28	59	93					
180.	1500	24	50	78	109	143			
200	1500	21	44	68	94	122	153	187	
220	1500	19	39	60	83	107	133	161	192
240	1500	17	35	54	74	95	118	142	168
260	1500	15	32	49	67	86	106	128	150
280	1500	14	29	45	62	79	97	116	136

Numbers in table are days to lose weight.

Table 3: Weight Loss Prediction for Men Ages 18–35

WEIGHT LOSS PREDICTION FOR MEN Ages 36-55
(Moderately Active During or After Working Hours)

Weight (lbs.)	Diet Calorie	Weight Loss Desired (lbs.)							
		10	20	30	40	50	60	70	80
140	1500	38							
160.	1500	31	66	105					
180.	1500	26	55	87	122	161			
200	1500	23	48	75	104	135	170	209	
220	1500	20	42	66	91	118	147	178	213
240	1500	18	38	59	81	104	129	156	185
260	1500	17	34	53	73	94	116	139	164
280	1500	15	32	49	67	85	105	126	148

Numbers in table are days to lose weight.

Table 4: Weight Loss Prediction for Men Ages 36–55

WEIGHT LOSS PREDICTION FOR MEN Ages 56-75
(Moderately Active During or After Working Hours)

Weight (lbs.)	Diet Calorie	Weight Loss Desired (lbs.)							
		10	20	30	40	50	60	70	80
140	1500	43							
160.	1500	34	73	117					
180.	1500	29	61	96	134	178			
200	1500	25	52	81	113	148	187	230	
220	1500	22	46	71	98	127	159	194	233
240	1500	20	41	63	87	112	139	168	200
260	1500	18	37	57	78	100	124	149	176
280	1500	16	34	52	71	91	112	134	158

Numbers in table are days to lose weight.

Table 5: Weight Loss Prediction for Men Ages 56–75

WEIGHT LOSS PREDICTION FOR WOMEN Ages: 18-35
(Moderately Active During or After Working Hours)

Present Weight (lbs.)	Diet Calories	Weight Loss Desired (lbs.)							
		5	10	15	20	30	40	50	60
120	1500	25	52	82					
130.	1500	22	45	70	97				
140.	1500	19	40	62	85	137			
160	1500	16	32	50	68	108	153	205	
180	1500	13	27	42	57	89	125	165	210
200	1500	12	24	36	49	76	106	138	174
220	1500	10	21	32	43	67	93	120	150
240	1500	9	19	29	39	60	82	106	132

Numbers in table are days to lose weight.

Table 6: Weight Loss Prediction for Women Ages 18–35

WEIGHT LOSS PREDICTION FOR WOMEN Ages: 36-55
(Moderately Active During or After Working Hours)

Present Weight (lbs.)	Diet Calories	Weight Loss Desired (lbs.)							
		5	10	15	20	30	40	50	60
120	1500	29	61						
130.	1500	25	52	81	113				
140.	1500	22	45	70	97	159			
160	1500	18	36	55	76	121	173	235	
180	1500	15	30	46	63	99	139	184	236
200	1500	13	26	40	54	84	117	153	193
220	1500	11	23	35	47	73	101	131	164
240	1500	10	20	31	42	65	89	115	143

Numbers in table are days to lose weight.

Table 7: Weight Loss Prediction for Women Ages 36–55

WEIGHT LOSS PREDICTION FOR WOMEN Ages: 56-75
(Moderately Active During or After Working Hours)

Present Weight (lbs.)	Diet Calories	Weight Loss Desired (lbs.)							
		5	10	15	20	30	40	50	60
120	1500	33	70	112					
130.	1500	28	58	92	129				
140.	1500	24	50	78	109	179			
160	1500	19	39	61	83	133	192	262	
180	1500	16	32	50	68	107	151	202	260
200	1500	14	28	42	58	90	126	165	209
220	1500	12	24	37	50	78	108	141	176
240	1500	11	22	33	45	69	95	123	153

Numbers in table are days to lose weight.
Table 8: Weight Loss Prediction for Women Ages 56–75

Expected Weight Loss

Assuming that the average man using this program is 36 to 55 years old and weighs 210 pounds, from Table 4 most **men should lose about 35 lbs in 80 days**. And assuming the average women is 36 to 55 years old and weighs 180 pounds, then from Table 7 most **women should lose about 25 lbs in 80 days**. Older and thinner people might lose a bit less; whereas younger and heavier people often lose much more.

Before You Begin

At the start of any weight loss program you should know where you stand, i.e., your current health status. **Everyone should at the very least have a medical assessment, or exam, before starting a weight loss diet.** Why? You need to make sure your health will allow you to lower your caloric intake and increase your physical activity. Depending on your age and state of health, the medical checkup may be as simple as a visit to a physician who is familiar with your medical history, or it may be a thorough physical exam.

The physician conducting the medical exam should be made aware of and should approve the specific weight loss diet you're planning. Additionally, because you are going to engage in physical activity in conjunction with this diet and especially if you have been totally inactive, or if you have or suspect you have cardiovascular disease or other health problems, or if you are obese, or if you are 40 or older, before embarking on the physical fitness portion of the program you probably should have a stress test supervised by a physician. Finally, your physician can tell you how much and what type of exercise is right for you, how much you should weigh, and prescribe a realistic weight- loss goal.

THE DIET PORTION

Most of us are busy – extremely busy under pressure to balance career, family, finances, a social life, friends, learning, and the list goes on and on. You know you should lose weight, but your life is just too hectic to plan and prepare low-calorie meals. *Maximum Weight Loss* can help. For those days when you don't have the time or energy to cook, choose from **45 daily no-cooking menus**. On the weekend, or whenever you have the time to cook, select from **45 daily cooking menus** complete with delicious easy to prepare recipes. In summary then, the *diet portion of the program* features:

- **45 Daily No-Cooking Menus**
- **45 Daily Cooking Menus**
- **48 Daily Cooking Recipes**

And every day on *Maximum Weight Loss* you get to decide to cook or not to cook and then you pick an appropriate daily menu from the large selection. But know that whether or not you cook you will be eating 1200 Calories and will lose the same amount of weight.

Using the No-Cooking Daily Menus

Let's look at No-Cooking **Daily Menu 2** on page 30. Most of the menu is obvious and easily understood. To find the line item **Microwaveable Soup #10** see **Appendix B** which lists microwaveable soups. In Appendix B on page 172, scan the left-most column until you find number 10. Immediately to the right is the soup for Day 2, Campbell's Healthy Request Classic Chicken Noodle soup.

To find the frozen entrée for No-Cooking **Daily Menu 2** first note that the allotment for the Day 2 frozen entrée is 200 Calories. Now go to **Appendix D** on page 176 which contains a list of about 150 frozen entrées arranged from lowest to highest in calorie content. In **Appendix D**, scroll down until you find the 200 Calorie frozen entrées. There are four entrées to choose from. Incidentally, because the diet calls for a ham sandwich for lunch, choose something other than a meat entrée for dinner, such as a 200 Calorie chicken or pasta frozen entrée. Remember variety is the key to a nutritious diet!

Using the Cooking Daily Menus

Go to Cooking **Daily Menu 1** on page 75. Again most of the menu is obvious and easily understood. To find the line item Recipe 1, go to page 121 which will bring you to the Recipe section. (Recipe 1 is Chicken with Peppers and Onions.)

Eat Smart

No single food can supply all the nutrients you need in the amounts you need. The most important factors in nutrition are variety, variety, variety! **Variety is the key to a nutritious diet.** As a means of setting strategies for food selection, the U.S. Department of Health and Human Services and the Department of Agriculture issue Dietary Guidelines every five years. The latest Dietary Guidelines describe a healthy diet as one that:
- Emphasizes fruits, vegetables, whole grains, and fat-free or low-fat milk products.
- Includes fish, poultry, lean meats, beans and nuts.
- Is low in saturated fats, trans fats, cholesterol, salt (sodium) and added sugars.

The latest guidelines encourage adults to consume a variety of nutrient-dense foods and beverages within their caloric needs. The afore mentioned U.S. government agencies recommend how much should be eaten from each of the basic food groups (i.e., from the fruit group, vegetable group, grains group, meat and beans group, milk group, and oils group) to meet your caloric goal – whether you are trying to lose weight or maintain weight. All this information and more can be found in *Eat Smart - U.S. Edition* published by NoPaperPress.

Even though most adults can get all the vitamins and minerals they need by merely consuming a variety of nutritious foods (from the fruit group, the vegetable group, the grains group, the meat and beans group, the milk group, and the oils group), many physicians recommend a daily multi-vitamin/mineral supplement – just in case you don't always eat the way you should.

No-Cooking: Big-Bowl Salad

The **No-Cooking Daily Menus** feature frozen entrees. A problem with nearly all frozen entrees is that they don't contain enough veggies. The solution is to have a "Big-Bowl Salad" at dinnertime with your frozen entrée. A typical "Big-Bowl Salad" is shown in the following photo.

To prepare a "Big-Bowl Salad" start with a relatively large soup bowl (with a volume of at least 24 ounces, or 3 cups). Add about 1½ cups of either green leaf lettuce, Romaine lettuce or a mesclun mix. Then add, as desired, veggies such as broccoli, celery, cucumber, onion, peppers, radish, spinach, tomato, or watercress, to make up the remaining 1½ cups, for a total of 3 cups. This vegetable combination will, on average, total about 100 Calories. You will be eating a "Big-Bowl Salad" almost every day at dinnertime. Remember that variety is the key to a nutritious diet. So be sure to vary the ingredients of the salad.

Top your "Big-Bowl Salad" with <u>2 tablespoons</u> of any light salad dressing available at your local supermarket that contains no more than 25 Calories per tablespoon. See some of my favorite light salad dressings below. Your "Big-Bowl Salad" with salad dressing will cost you roughly 150 Calories but will be packed with lots of health-giving vitamins, minerals and fiber.

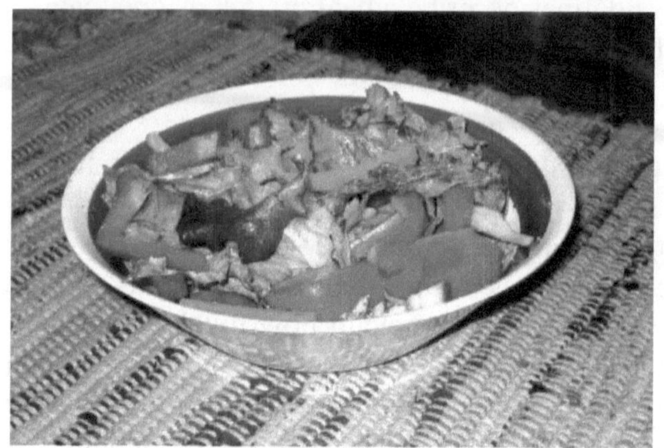
Big-Bowl Salad

Cooking: Have a Tossed Salad

One of the dinner mainstays in the **Cooking Daily Menus** is a tossed salad." To prepare your "Tossed Salad" start with a bowl that has a volume of about 16 ounces, or 2 cups. First add about 1 cup of either green leaf lettuce, Romaine lettuce or a mesclun mix. Then add at least a half cup of other veggies such as broccoli, celery, cucumber, peppers, spinach, watercress, or tomatoes. This vegetable combination will, on average, total something like 45 Calories.

You'll be eating a "Tossed Salad" just about every day at dinnertime. Once again, variety is the key to a nutritious diet. So vary the ingredients of the salad.

Top your "Tossed Salad" with <u>1½ tablespoons of any light salad dressing</u> available at your local supermarket that contains no more than 25 Calories per tablespoon.

Your "Tossed Salad" with salad dressing will cost you roughly 85 Calories but will be packed with lots of health-giving vitamins, minerals and fiber.

Recommended Salad Dressings

For your consideration, here are some of my favorite light salad dressings. All have a maximum of 25 Calories per tablespoon.

- **Ken's Steakhouse Fat Free Raspberry**
- **Kraft Light Done Right House Italian**
- **Wishbone Just 2 Good Honey Dijon**
- **Newman's Lighten Up Balsamic Vinaigrette**

About Bread

First understand that bread, more specifically whole-grain breads, are good sources of complex carbohydrates and dietary fiber, as well as several B vitamins (thiamin, riboflavin, niacin, and folate), vitamin E, and minerals (iron, magnesium and selenium). In recent years, however, sliced bread loaves have gotten larger, as have the bread slices inside these loaves. Just a few years ago the standard slice of bread contained about 65 to 70 Calories – now most are 100 plus Calories.

Maximum Weight Loss **requires whole-grain bread at 70 Calories per slice.** Quite a few bakers sell thin sliced or "light" sliced bread. The difficult part is finding a whole grain thin sliced or "light" bread (with about 70 Calories per slice). Whatever the brand, make sure the first word in the Ingredients list is "whole." "Pepperidge Farm Small Slice 100% Whole Wheat" is a good choice. It's whole grain, has 70 Calories per slice and it tastes good too.

Important Notes

1) Coffee or tea may be caffeinated or decaf . If desired, skim milk and a sugar substitute may be added to coffee or tea. And soy or almond milk may be used instead of cow's milk.

2) Fried eggs or scrambled eggs should be cooked in a pan coated with a non-stick cooking spray. Hard-boiled eggs may be substituted for fried, scrambled or soft-boiled eggs.

3) Cereals should be whole grain and unsweetened. At the top of the list are Old-fashioned Oatmeal, Wheatena and Shredded Wheat. Among other reasonably healthy choices are Cheerios, Wheat Chex, Wheaties, some Kashi cereals and Farina. When blueberries are in season, you may **add blueberries instead of raisins** to your cereal. (Substitution ratio = 2 blueberries per raisin.)

4) Bread may be either plain or toasted whole grain, such as whole grain, whole rye or pumpernickel. Look for whole grain varieties that contain 70 Calories per slice. If desired, bread may be sprayed with a zero-calorie butter substitute. NO BUTTER!

5) When soup in a microwaveable bowl is specified, eat only one serving (8 ounces) unless otherwise noted. (Microwaveable bowls usually contain about two servings.)

6) Use freely as desired: clear unsweetened coffee, clear unsweetened tea, water, seltzer water and any diet soda, clear soups without fat, bouillon, and seasonings such as mustard, cinnamon, dill, herbs, red and black pepper, curry, vinegar, lemon juice and sections, and dill and sour pickles.

7) Use only lean cuts of meat trimmed of all visible fat. Poultry should be limited to chicken or turkey breasts (white meat only and skinless).

8) When canned tuna or salmon is specified, use only fish packed in water.

9) When the diet calls for turkey bacon, make sure the brand you buy has no more than 35 Calories per slice.

10) An unlimited amount of green salad may be eaten, but the salad dressing should be as specified.

11) If it's more convenient, any food item may be moved to any part of the day and combined with any meal or snack.

12) Although it's recommended that you follow the diet days as specified, it's fine to occasionally skip a day and/or pick and choose the days you prefer. (Nutritionally, each day stands on its own.)

13) **Take a daily multi-vitamin/mineral supplement**. This is important when you're on a diet – as a kind of insurance policy.

THE WORKOUT PORTION

In order to qualify for as moderately active, you must exercise at least six days a week! Be careful and approach this portion of *Maximum Weight Loss* cautiously - especially if you have been relatively inactive.

You will be walking four days and exercising with dumbbells two days a week. Your walking objective is 10,000 steps - which has been shown to promote weight loss and to improve your cardio-vascular system. The dumbbell lifts build muscle and speed up your metabolism.

Program: Walk two days then use the dumbbells for one day. Repeat this routine for the following three days. Then rest on the seventh day.

In summary: Day 1) Walk, Day 2) Walk, Day 3) Dumbbell workout, Day 4) Walk, Day 5) Walk, Day 6) Dumbbell workout, Day 7) Rest.

More on Walking

Sedentary people only take about 2,000 to 3,000 steps a day. But a Harvard University study has shown that 6,000 steps a day correlate with lower death rates in men, and that 8,000 to 10,000 steps per day promote weight loss. And these health and weight management benefits don't oblige you to walk continuously until you accrue the required number of steps. Rather, all steps throughout the day to wherever and whenever count toward your daily total. Because 8,000 to 10,000 steps a day may not be achievable by some people, particularly by those who are elderly or sedentary, rather than insisting on a blanket 10,000 steps per day, at the beginning of the program your stepping goal should be based on your baseline steps plus an increment of additional steps. (Your baseline being the number of steps taken in an average day.)

A pedometer keeps track of your steps. And a study by the American College of Sports Medicine found that participants who used pedometers were motivated to add about 2,000 steps to their daily routine. To start a stepping program, buy a pedometer. Wear the pedometer for a week and determine the number of steps you take on an average day. This is your baseline. Then add the equivalent of half an hour of walking to your day, or
roughly 2,500 extra steps per day. For example, consider a woman who uses a pedometer and notes that on an average day she accumulates 3,500 steps. Her goal should be to add the equivalent of a half hour of walking to her day, or roughly 2,500 more steps per day, for a daily total of 6,000 steps.

There are many little ways to add steps to your day, such as taking stairs rather than an elevator, parking further from your destination, pacing as you talk on the telephone, marching-in-place for a minute once every hour – and of course taking short walks whenever you can. So get a pedometer, or a Fitbit, or use a pedometer app on your smart phone. Get off the couch and step out!

Dumbbell Exercises

If you are a beginner it's probably worthwhile to start by joining a health club, where you can get professional instruction on the proper use of exercise equipment, from dumbbells to rowing machines, and where you can compare different exercise routines. Another possibility is to hire a personal trainer for a couple of sessions to get you started on a program personalized to your fitness level and to teach you correct exercise techniques.

Of all the many strength-building options, this writer prefers free weights (actually dumbbells) because they can be used at home. Working out at home has some significant advantages. First, your workout takes less time because you don't have to drive back and forth to a health club; second, you have the flexibility of dividing your workout into small time segments to fit your day, whenever you have time, such as when the baby is napping, and of course working out at home is certainly less expensive.

You can workout in a bedroom, basement, garage, attic – anywhere you have extra space. A set of variable (adjustable) weight dumbbells and a small weight bench don't take up much room and are all you need for a home-based gym. (Bear in mind, **knowledge and the discipline to work out regularly are far more important than fancy equipment**.) Before investing in a set of weights and a bench, however, it may still be worthwhile to start by joining a health club. At a health club you can get expert instruction on the use of free weights. And you may find that you actually prefer to workout at a club. But if you do decide to opt for the convenience of a home-based gym, that would be the time to purchase a pair of variable-weight dumbbells and a strong weight bench for home use. Rather than an entire set of weights, initially purchase just enough dumbbell weight so that you can do a military press five times.

The seven dumbbell exercises that follow comprise a total-body workout, suitable for beginners, that involve all the major muscle groups. When done consecutively without stopping a series of exercises is called a circuit. To start, use the same dumbbell weight for all the exercises, a weight that allows you to do about 10 repetitions of the most difficult exercise in the circuit. For the first week do one circuit per training session. Your goal should be two circuits per session, which should take you about 20 minutes (with a two to three-minute rest between circuits). When you are comfortable at this level you are ready to increase the dumbbell weight – but by no more than roughly 10 percent (or one pound minimum). Again, work up to a dumbbell weight so you can perform 10 to 15 repetitions of each exercise in the circuit. The seven exercises are described and illustrated in on the following pages.

a) <u>Bench Press</u>: With your head and back on the bench, hold a dumbbell in each hand to the side of your shoulders, palms facing each other. Slowly raise the dumbbells extending your arms above your shoulders. Pause, then lower the dumbbells down to the starting position. The bench press primarily works your pectorals, triceps and deltoids.

b) <u>One–Arm Dumbbell Row</u>: Hold a dumbbell in your right hand, palm facing toward your right thigh. Stand to the right of your weight bench and place your left knee on the bench. Support yourself by putting your left hand on the bench. (Flex your right knee slightly and lean forward so your back is almost parallel to the floor.) Slowly pull your right arm up until your upper arm is parallel to the floor. (Keep your right arm close to your torso.) Pause and lower your right arm to the starting position. After you complete a set, stand to the left of the bench and repeat the exercise with the dumbbell in your left hand. Rows mainly work your latissimus dorsi and rhomboid muscles in your back.

c) <u>Seated Shoulder Press</u>: From a seated position, hold a dumbbell in each hand to the side of your shoulders, palms facing forward. Slowly raise the weights over your head until your arms are straight. Pause, then lower the dumbbells to the starting position. The shoulder press mainly exercises your deltoids, trapezius, triceps, latissimus dorsi and rhomboid muscles.

d) <u>Curls for Biceps</u>: Stand with a dumbbell in each hand, your arms hanging loosely, with your palms to the side your thighs and facing straight ahead. Keep your elbows tucked into your side and slowly lift the dumbbells until they are approximately shoulder high. Pause and lower the dumbbells to the starting
position. Curls chiefly work your biceps.

e) <u>Tricep Extension (or Kickback)</u>: With a dumbbell in your right hand, assume the same initial position as in the one-arm dumbbell row. Slowly move your right arm rearward until it is nearly parallel to the floor. Pause and then return the dumbbell to the starting position. Kickbacks work your triceps and deltoids.

f) <u>Front Squats</u>: Stand with a dumbbell in each hand, to the side of your shoulders, palms facing each other (inward). Slowly bend your knees and lower your body until your thighs are almost parallel to the floor. Try to keep your heels on the floor. Pause and gradually raise your body by straightening your knees. Squats work your gluteus, quadriceps and hamstrings.

g) <u>Curl for Abs</u>: This is not a weight lifting exercise but is a useful part of any routine. Lie face up on a floor mat with your hands folded over your chest and your legs bent. Keeping your feet flat on the mat, slowly curl your torso up and toward your thighs until your shoulder blades are off the mat. Pause, then return to the starting position. This exercise works your rectus abdominis muscles – your abs.

Bench Press

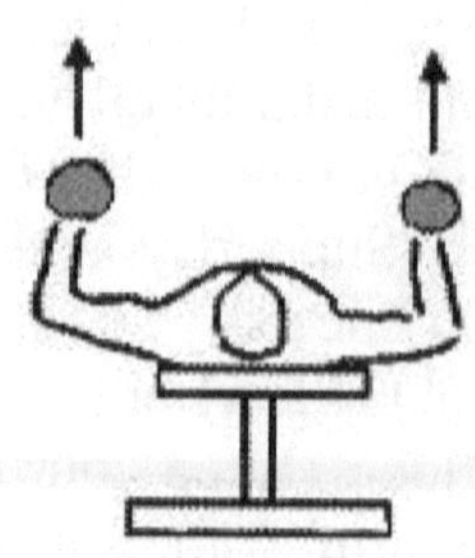 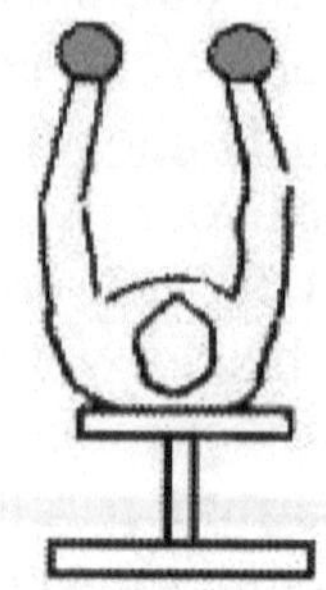

One-Arm Row

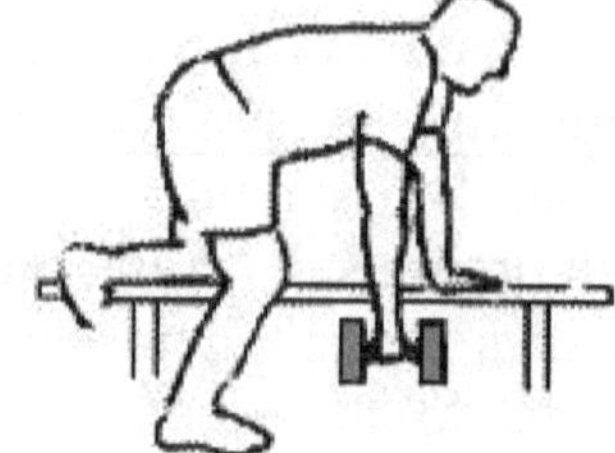 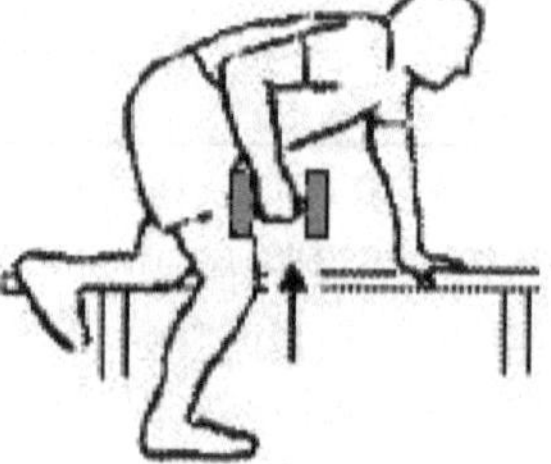

**Seated
Shoulder
Press**

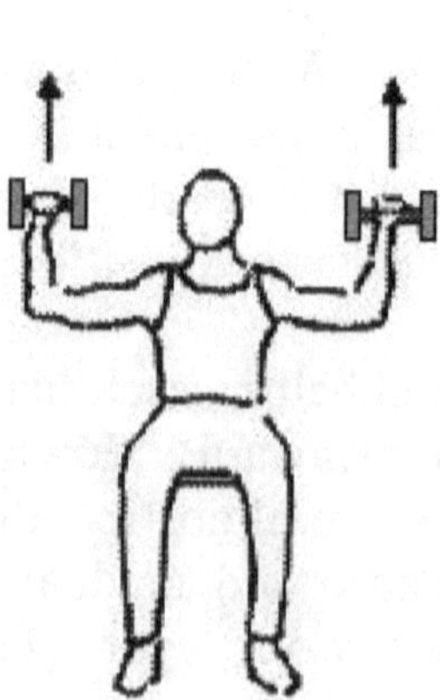 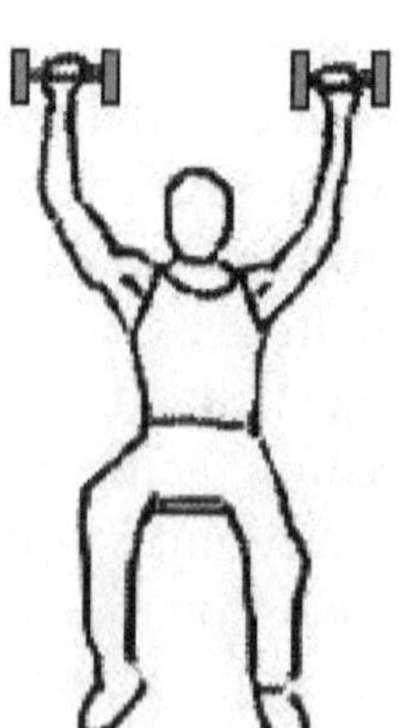

Bicep Curls

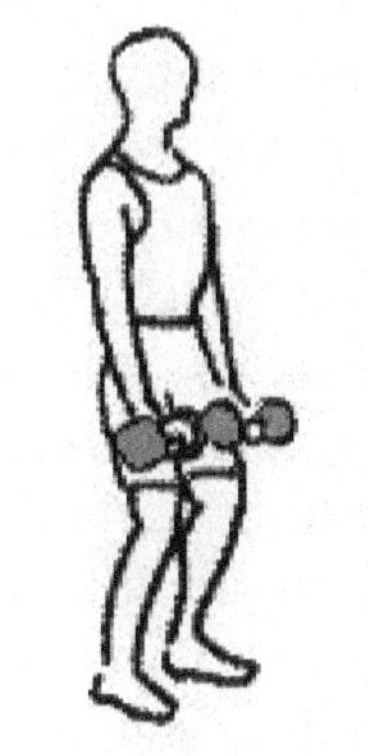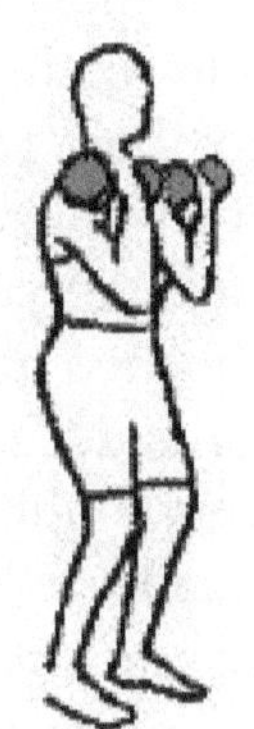

Tricep Extension

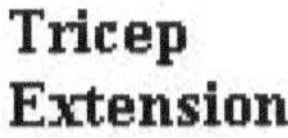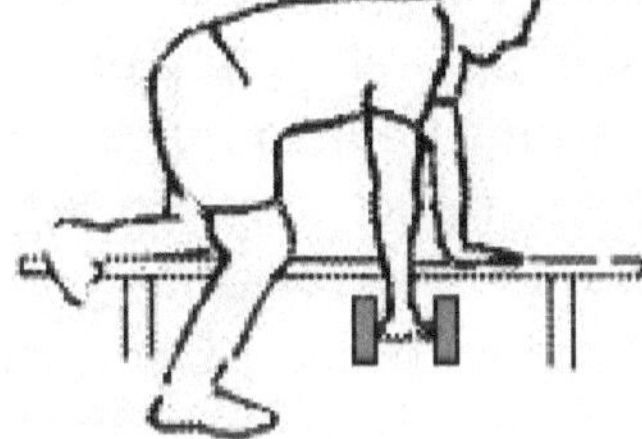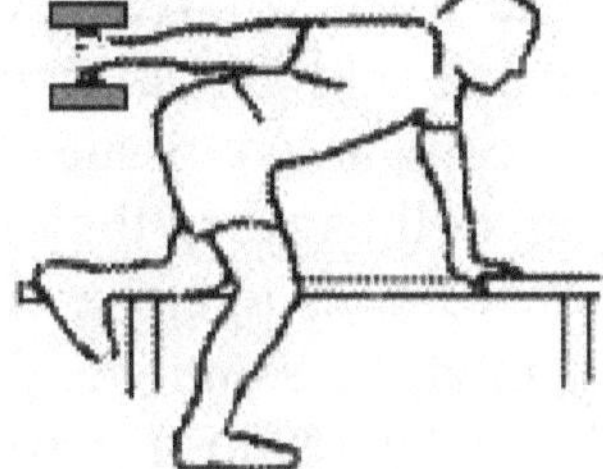

Front Squat

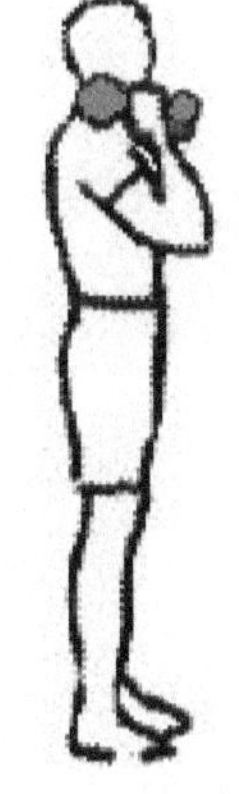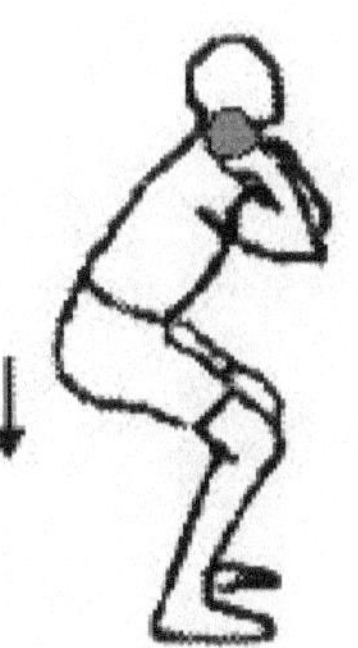

Curl for Abs

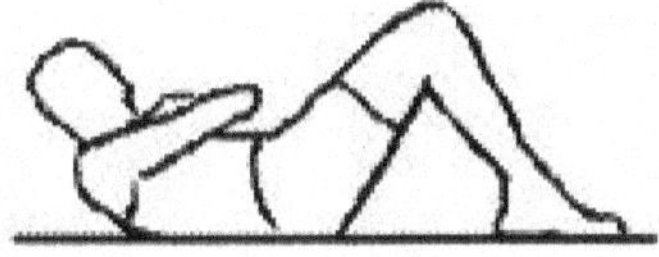

Keep It Off

Within five years, more than 60 percent of all dieters regain every pound they have lost. Why? In most cases it's because after losing weight most people eventually revert to their pre-diet eating and exercising habits, and this inevitably leads to their regaining the weight they lost – and often more. Obviously after a diet you weigh less. The fact is the less you weigh, the less you need to eat to sustain your lower weight.

A study, published in the *Annals of Internal Medicine*, that followed 4,000 people for three decades suggests that in the long term 60 percent of the people became overweight. Interestingly, half of the men and women in the study, who had made it well into adulthood without a weight problem, ultimately also became overweight and a third actually became obese. The point being that you must continually watch your weight because we are all at risk of becoming overweight.

And when you reach your mid to late twenties, you slowly start to lose muscle and add fat as part of the natural aging process. But muscle is metabolically active tissue. This means your muscles use calories when they work, as well as when they repair and refuel. Fat, on the other hand, requires very few calories to exist. This is one of the reasons you need fewer calories to remain at the same weight as you get older. The quantity of food energy required to <u>maintain</u> a particular weight is again a function of gender, age, weight and activity level, as is clearly shown in the following Weight Maintenance Table.

Maintenance Calories for Moderately Active People

Weight Lbs.	Women			Men		
	18 - 35	36 - 55	56 - 75	18 - 35	36 - 55	56 - 75
110	2170	2085	2008			
115	2230	2144	2065			
120	2289	2201	2121	2434	2304	2201
125	2347	2258	2176	2495	2363	2258
130	2405	2314	2231	2556	2421	2314
135	2463	2370	2286	2615	2479	2370
140	2519	2425	2340	2674	2536	2425
145	2575	2480	2393	2733	2592	2480
150	2631	2534	2446	2791	2648	2534
160	2741	2642	2551	2905	2759	2642
170	2850	2748	2655	3018	2867	2748
180	2957	2852	2757	3129	2975	2852
190	3062	2955	2858	3239	3081	2955
200	3166	3057	2957	3347	3185	3057
210	3270	3158	3056	3454	3289	3158
220	3372	3258	3154	3560	3391	3258
230	3473	3357	3251	3664	3493	3357
240	3573	3455	3347	3768	3593	3455
250	3672	3552	3442	3871	3692	3552
260				3972	3792	3648
270				4073	3890	3744
280				4173	3987	3839

Table 9: Weight Maintenance Calories per Day

From Table 9, note that for the same age and weight women need fewer weight maintenance calories than men - to neither gain nor lose weight. Also, as you lose weight your weight maintenance calorie needs decrease! For more on this, once you reach your weight goal, read ***Weight Maintenance - U.S. Edition*** (published NoPaperPress).

No-Cooking
Daily Meal Plans

No-Cooking Daily Menu 1

BREAKFAST	Calories	Totals
Fresh or frozen strawberries (½ cup)	25	
Kashi Go Lean Waffles* (2)	150	
Morningstar Breakfast Sausage Link*	80	
Light Syrup (2 Tbsp)	50	
Coffee (See Notes - page 21)	10	315 Cal
SNACK		
Yogurt (4 oz, non-fat any flavor)**	60	
Coffee or tea	10	70 Cal
** Such as Dannon Lite & Fit. Buy 32 oz container & use 4 oz.		
LUNCH		
Ham (2 oz) with mustard on 2 slices rye bread	300	
Laughing Cow Light Cheese (1 wedge)	35	
Fresh fruit in season (apple, peach, etc)	70	
Coffee or tea	10	415 Cal
SNACK		
Coffee or tea	10	10 Cal
DINNER		
Frozen Entrée (Appendix D - page 176)	200	
"Big-Bowl Salad" (See Dressings - page 20)	150	
Whole-grain bread (1 slice) (See page 21)	70	
Fresh fruit in season (apple, peach, etc)	70	
Water	0	490 Cal
SNACK		
Skinny Cow Ice Cream Sandwich*	160	
Coffee or tea	10	170 Cal
* If unavailable an equivalent dessert.		1500 Cal

No-Cooking Daily Menu 2

BREAKFAST	Calories	Totals
Orange juice (½ cup)	50	
Wheaties (¾ cup) + ½ cup skim milk + ½ banana	190	
Whole-grain toast (1 slice)	70	
Coffee	10	320 Cal
SNACK		
Fresh fruit in season (apple, peach, etc)	70	
Coffee or tea	10	80 Cal
LUNCH		
Soup (Appendix B - page 172)	110	
String cheese (1 piece, any brand)*	80	
Whole-grain bread (1 slice)	70	
Coffee or tea	10	270 Cal
* Maximum of 80 Calories		
SNACK		
Coffee or tea	10	10 Cal
DINNER		
Frozen Entrée (Appendix D - page 176)	300	
"Big-Bowl Salad" (See page 20)	150	
Fresh fruit in season (pear, peach, etc)	70	
Water with lemon wedge	15	605 Cal
SNACK		
Popcorn Mini Bag**	110	
Coffee or tea	10	120 Cal
** Such as Orville Redenbacher's Smart Pop		1505 Cal

No-Cooking Daily Menu 3

BREAKFAST	Calories	Totals
Grapefruit (½)	75	
Scrambled egg (Notes - page 21)	80	
Turkey bacon (1 slice) (Notes)	35	
Whole-grain toast (1 slice)	70	
Coffee	10	270 Cal
SNACK		
Yogurt (4 oz, non-fat any flavor)	60	
Coffee or tea	10	70 Cal
LUNCH		
Soup (Appendix B - page 172)	130	
String cheese (1 piece, any brand)	80	
Fresh fruit in season (pear, peach, etc)	70	
Coffee or tea	10	290 Cal
SNACK		
Handful unsalted mixed nuts	100	
Coffee or tea	10	110 Cal
DINNER		
Frozen Entrée (Appendix D - page 176)	270	
"Big-Bowl Salad"	150	
Whole-grain bread (1 slice)	70	
Fresh fruit in season (apple, peach, etc)	70	
Water with lemon wedge	15	575 Cal
SNACK		
Kashi TLC Crunchy Granola Bar*	180	
Coffee or tea	10	190 Cal
* If unavailable an equivalent dessert.		1505 Cal

No-Cooking Daily Menu 4

BREAKFAST	Calories	Totals
Grapefruit (½)	75	
Cheerios (1 cup) + ½ cup skim milk + about 15 raisins*	190	
Coffee	10	275 Cal
SNACK		
Handful unsalted mixed nuts	100	
Coffee or tea	10	110 Cal
LUNCH		
Cottage cheese (1 cup low fat)	180	
Fresh fruit in season (apple, plum, etc)	70	
Small whole-grain roll	80	
Coffee or tea	10	340 Cal
SNACK		
Kashi TLC Crunchy Granola Bar	180	
Coffee or tea	10	190 Cal
DINNER		
Frozen Entrée (Appendix D - page 176)	270	
"Big-Bowl Salad"	150	
Whole-grain bread (1 slice)	70	
Water with lemon wedge	15	500 Cal
SNACK		
Fresh fruit in season (apple, plum, etc)	70	
Coffee or tea	10	80 Cal
* See Notes - page 13 re substituting blueberries for raisins.		1495 Cal

No-Cooking Daily Menu 5

BREAKFAST	Calories	Totals
Cantaloupe (½ medium)	50	
Fried eggs (2)	160	
Toasted raisin bread (1 slice)	75	
Coffee	10	295 Cal
SNACK		
Yogurt (4 oz, non-fat any flavor)	60	
Coffee or tea	10	70 Cal
LUNCH		
Salad (3 oz canned tuna, 1 tsp Evoo, onions, celery)	175	
String cheese (1 piece, any brand - 80 Cal max)	80	
Rye bread (1 slice)	70	
Diet soda or water	0	325 Cal
SNACK		
Fresh fruit in season (apple, peach, etc)	70	
Coffee or tea	10	80 Cal
DINNER		
Frozen Entrée (Appendix D - page 176)	190	
"Big-Bowl Salad"	150	
Small whole-grain roll	80	
Glass of wine (4 oz)	100	
Water with lemon wedge	15	555 Cal
SNACK		
Skinny Cow Ice Cream Sandwich**	160	
Coffee or tea	10	170 Cal
** If unavailable an equivalent dessert.		1495 Cal

No-Cooking Daily Menu 6

BREAKFAST	Calories	Totals
Tomato juice (½ cup)	**20**	
Shredded Wheat (1 cup) + ½ cup skim milk + ½ banana	**265**	
Coffee	**10**	**295 Cal**
SNACK		
Yogurt (4 oz, non-fat any flavor)	**60**	
Coffee or tea	**10**	**70 Cal**
LUNCH		
Ham & Cheddar*	**270**	
Fresh fruit in season (pear, plum, etc)	**70**	
Diet soda or water	**0**	**340 Cal**
* Hot Pockets Wrap or if unavailable and equivalent food.		
SNACK		
Coffee or tea	**10**	**10 Cal**
DINNER		
Frozen Entrée (Appendix D - page 176)	**300**	
"Big-Bowl Salad"	**150**	
Whole-grain bread (1 slice)	**70**	
Fresh blueberries, cherries or grapes (1 cup)	**100**	
Water with lemon wedge	**15**	**635 Cal**
SNACK		
Kashi TLC Chewy Granola Bar*	**140**	
Coffee or tea	**10**	**150 Cal**
* If unavailable an equivalent food.		**1500 Cal**

No-Cooking Daily Menu 7

BREAKFAST	Calories	Totals
Orange juice (½ cup)	50	
Wheat Chex (¾ cup) + ½ cup skim milk + ½ banana	250	
Coffee	10	310 Cal
SNACK		
Fresh fruit in season (apple, peach, etc)	70	
Coffee or tea	10	80 Cal
LUNCH		
Soup (Appendix B - page 172)	140	
String cheese (1 piece, any brand)	80	
Whole-grain bread (1 slice)	70	
Coffee or tea	10	300 Cal
SNACK		
Handful unsalted mixed nuts	100	
Coffee or tea	10	110 Cal
DINNER		
Frozen Entrée (Appendix D - page 176)	270	
"Big-Bowl Salad"	150	
Whole-grain bread (1 slice)	70	
Fresh fruit in season (apple, peach, etc)	70	
Water with lemon wedge	15	575 Cal
SNACK		
Popcorn Mini Bag	110	
Coffee or tea	10	120 Cal
		1495 Cal

No-Cooking Daily Menu 8

BREAKFAST	Calories	Totals
Orange juice (½ cup)	50	
Kashi Go Lean Waffles (2)	150	
Morningstar Breakfast Sausage Link	80	
Light Syrup (2 Tbsp)	50	
Coffee	10	340 Cal
SNACK		
Yogurt (4 oz, non-fat any flavor)	60	
Coffee or tea	10	70 Cal
LUNCH		
Subway 6" (Ham, Cheese +veggies)*	260	
Fresh fruit in season (peach, plum, etc)	70	
Coffee or tea	10	340 Cal
* Half whole-grain roll		
SNACK		
Handful unsalted mixed nuts	100	
Coffee or tea	10	110 Cal
DINNER		
Frozen Entrée (Appendix D - page 176)	230	
"Big-Bowl Salad"	150	
Whole-grain bread (1 slice)	70	
Water with lemon wedge	15	465 Cal
SNACK		
Skinny Cow Ice Cream Sandwich	160	
Coffee or tea	10	170 Cal
		1495 Cal

No-Cooking Daily Menu 9

BREAKFAST	Calories	Totals
Grapefruit (½)	75	
Scrambled egg	80	
Whole-grain toast (1 slice)	70	
Coffee	10	235 Cal
SNACK		
Yogurt (4 oz, non-fat any flavor)	60	
Coffee or tea	10	70 Cal
LUNCH		
Soup (Appendix B - page 172)	200	
Laughing Cow Light Cheese (2 wedges)	70	
Fresh fruit in season (apple, plum, etc)	70	
Coffee or tea	10	360 Cal
SNACK		
Handful unsalted mixed nuts	100	
Coffee or tea	10	110 Cal
DINNER		
Frozen Entrée (Appendix D - page 176)	300	
"Big-Bowl Salad"	150	
Whole-grain bread (1 slice)	70	
Fresh fruit in season (apple, plum, etc)	70	
Water with lemon wedge	15	605 Cal
SNACK		
Popcorn Mini Bag	110	
Coffee or tea	10	120 Cal
		1500 Cal

No-Cooking Daily Menu 10

BREAKFAST	Calories	Totals
Fresh sliced orange	75	
Cheerios (1 cup) + ½ cup skim milk + about 15 raisins	190	
Whole-grain toast (1 slice)	70	
Coffee	10	345 Cal
SNACK		
Handful unsalted mixed nuts	100	
Coffee or tea	10	110 Cal
LUNCH		
Cottage cheese (1 cup low fat)	180	
Fresh fruit in season (apple, plum, etc)	70	
Small whole-grain roll	80	
Coffee or tea	10	340 Cal
SNACK		
Kashi TLC Chewy Granola Bar	140	
Coffee or tea	10	150 Cal
DINNER		
Frozen Entrée (Appendix D - page 176)	220	
"Big-Bowl Salad"	150	
Yogurt (4 oz, non-fat any flavor)	60	
Hot or iced tea	10	440 Cal
SNACK		
Popcorn Mini Bag	110	
Coffee or tea	10	120 Cal
		1505 Cal

No-Cooking Daily Menu 11

BREAKFAST	Calories	Totals
Grapefruit (½)	75	
Scrambled egg	80	
Turkey bacon (1 slice)	35	
Whole-grain toast (1 slice)	70	
Coffee	10	270 Cal
SNACK		
Fresh fruit in season (apple, plum, etc)	70	
Coffee or tea	10	80 Cal
LUNCH		
Soup (Appendix B - page 172)	220	
Laughing Cow Light Cheese (1 wedge)	35	
Small whole-grain roll	80	
Coffee or tea	10	345 Cal
SNACK		
Yogurt (4 oz, non-fat any flavor)	60	
Coffee or tea	10	70 Cal
DINNER		
Frozen Entrée (Appendix D - page 176)	330	
"Big-Bowl Salad"	150	
Fresh fruit in season (apple, peach, etc)	70	
Water with lemon wedge	15	565 Cal
SNACK		
Skinny Cow Ice Cream Sandwich	160	
Coffee or tea	10	170 Cal
		1500 Cal

No-Cooking Daily Menu 12

BREAKFAST	Calories	Totals
Orange juice (½ cup)	50	
Shredded Wheat (1 cup) + ½ cup skim milk + ½ banana	260	
Coffee	10	320 Cal
SNACK		
Fresh fruit in season (apple, plum, etc)	70	
Coffee or tea	10	80 Cal
LUNCH		
Peanut butter (2 Tbsp) on 2 slices whole-grain bread	340	
Skim milk (6 oz)	70	
Fresh fruit in season (apple, plum, etc)	70	
Water	0	480 Cal
SNACK		
100-Calorie Pack Cookies*	100	
Coffee or tea	10	110 Cal
DINNER		
Frozen Entrée (Appendix D - page 176)	200	
"Big-Bowl Salad"	150	
Hot or iced tea	10	340 Cal
SNACK		
Kashi TLC Chewy Granola Bar	140	
Coffee or tea	10	150 Cal
* Such as Nabisco Oreo/Chips Ahoy/etc		1500 Cal

No-Cooking Daily Menu 13

BREAKFAST	Calories	Totals
Fresh sliced orange	75	
Wheaties (¾ cup) + ½ cup skim milk + ½ banana	190	
Whole grain toast (1 slice)	70	
Coffee	10	345 Cal
SNACK		
Fresh fruit in season (apple, plum, etc)	70	
Coffee or tea	10	80 Cal
LUNCH		
Soup (Appendix B - page 172)	100	
String cheese (1 piece, any brand)	80	
Small whole-grain roll	80	
Coffee or tea	10	270 Cal
SNACK		
Handful unsalted mixed nuts	100	
Coffee or tea	10	110 Cal
DINNER		
Frozen Entrée (Appendix D - page 176)	350	
"Big-Bowl Salad"	150	
Fresh fruit in season (apple, plum, etc)	70	
Water with lemon wedge	15	565 Cal
SNACK		
Popcorn Mini Bag	110	
Coffee or tea	10	120 Cal
		1490 Cal

No-Cooking Daily Menu 14

BREAKFAST	Calories	Totals
Orange juice (½ cup)	50	
Wheat Chex (¾ cup) + ½ cup skim milk + ½ banana	250	
Coffee	10	310 Cal
SNACK		
Yogurt (4 oz, non-fat any flavor)	60	
Coffee or tea	10	70 Cal
LUNCH		
Ham & Cheddar*	270	
Small bunch of grapes	50	
Diet soda or water	0	320 Cal
* Hot Pockets Wrap or an equivalent food.		
SNACK		
Handful unsalted mixed nuts	100	
Coffee or tea	10	110 Cal
DINNER		
Frozen Entrée (Appendix D - page 176)	220	
"Big-Bowl Salad"	150	
Whole-grain bread (1 slice)	70	
Fresh fruit in season (apple, peach, etc)	70	
Water with lemon wedge	15	525 Cal
SNACK		
Skinny Cow Ice Cream Sandwich	160	
Coffee or tea	10	170 Cal
		1505 Cal

No-Cooking Daily Menu 15

BREAKFAST	Calories	Totals
Cantaloupe (½ medium)	50	
Scrambled egg	80	
Turkey bacon (2 slices)	70	
Toasted raisin bread (1 slice)	75	
Coffee	10	285 Cal
SNACK		
Yogurt (4 oz, non-fat any flavor)	60	
Coffee or tea	10	70 Cal
LUNCH		
Soup (Appendix B - page 172)	170	
String cheese (1 piece, any brand)	80	
Nature Valley Crunchy Granola bar	95	
Coffee or tea	10	355 Cal
SNACK		
Handful unsalted mixed nuts	100	
Coffee or tea	10	110 Cal
DINNER		
Frozen Entrée (Appendix D - page 176)	270	
"Big-Bowl Salad"	150	
Whole-grain bread (1 slice)	70	
Fresh fruit in season (apple, plum, etc)	70	
Water	0	560 Cal
SNACK		
Popcorn Mini Bag	110	
Coffee or tea	10	120 Cal
		1500 Cal

No-Cooking Daily Menu 16

BREAKFAST	Calories	Totals
Grapefruit (½)	75	
Cheerios (1 cup) + ½ cup skim milk + about 15 raisins	190	
Coffee	10	275 Cal
SNACK		
Handful unsalted mixed nuts	100	
Coffee or tea	10	110 Cal
LUNCH		
Cottage cheese (1 cup low fat)	180	
Fresh fruit in season (apple, plum, etc)	70	
Small whole-grain roll	80	
Coffee or tea	10	340 Cal
SNACK		
Kashi TLC Chewy Granola Bar	140	
Coffee or tea	10	150 Cal
DINNER		
Frozen Entrée (Appendix D - page 176)	210	
"Big-Bowl Salad"	150	
Whole-grain bread (1 slice)	70	
Fresh fruit in season (apple, plum, etc)	70	
Water	0	500 Cal
SNACK		
Popcorn Mini Bag	110	
Coffee or tea	10	120 Cal
		1495 Cal

No-Cooking Daily Menu 17

BREAKFAST	Calories	Totals
Grapefruit (½)	75	
Fried egg	80	
Whole-grain toast (2 slices)	140	
Coffee	10	305 Cal
SNACK		
Yogurt (4 oz, non-fat any flavor)	60	
Coffee or tea	10	70 Cal
LUNCH		
Salad (3 oz canned tuna, 1 tsp Evoo, onions, celery)	175	
Rye bread (1 slice)	70	
Hot or iced tea	10	255 Cal
SNACK		
Handful unsalted mixed nuts	100	
Coffee or tea	10	110 Cal
DINNER		
Frozen Entrée (Appendix D - page 176)	330	
"Big-Bowl Salad"	150	
Fresh fruit in season (pear, plum, etc)	70	
Water with lemon wedge	15	565 Cal
SNACK		
Kashi TLC Crunchy Granola Bar	180	
Coffee or tea	10	190 Cal
		1495 Cal

No-Cooking Daily Menu 18

BREAKFAST	Calories	Totals
Tomato juice (½ cup)	20	
Shredded Wheat (1 cup) + ½ cup skim milk + ½ banana	260	
Coffee	10	290 Cal
SNACK		
Yogurt (4 oz, non-fat any flavor)	60	60 Cal
LUNCH		
Chicken Bacon Ranch*	270	
Fresh fruit in season (apple, plum, etc)	70	
Diet soda or water	0	340 Cal
* Hot Pockets (wrap) or an equivalent food.		
SNACK		
Handful unsalted mixed nuts	100	
Coffee or tea	10	110 Cal
DINNER		
Frozen Entrée (Appendix D - page 176)	270	
"Big-Bowl Salad"	150	
Whole-grain bread (1 slice)	70	
Fresh fruit in season (apple, plum, etc)	70	
Water	0	560 Cal
SNACK		
Kashi TLC Chewy Granola Bar	140	140 Cal
		1500 Cal

BREAKFAST	Calories	Totals
Cantaloupe (½ medium)	50	
Wheat Chex (¾ cup) + ½ cup skim milk + ½ banana	250	
Coffee	10	310 Cal
SNACK		
Fresh fruit in season (peach, plum, etc)	70	
Coffee or tea	10	80 Cal
LUNCH		
Soup (Appendix B - page 172)	150	
String cheese (1 piece, any brand)	80	
Small whole-grain roll	80	
Coffee or tea	10	320 Cal
SNACK		
Handful unsalted mixed nuts	100	
Coffee or tea	10	110 Cal
DINNER		
Frozen Entrée (Appendix D - page 176)	260	
"Big-Bowl Salad"	150	
Whole-grain bread (1 slice)	70	
Fresh fruit in season (peach, plum, etc)	70	
Water with lemon wedge	15	565 Cal
SNACK		
Popcorn Mini Bag	110	110 Cal
		1505 Cal

No-Cooking Daily Menu 20

BREAKFAST	Calories	Totals
Fresh or frozen strawberries (½ cup)	25	
Kashi Go Lean Waffles (2)	150	
Morningstar Breakfast Sausage Link	80	
Light Syrup (2 Tbsp)	50	
Coffee	10	315 Cal
SNACK		
Yogurt (4 oz, non-fat any flavor)	60	
Coffee or tea	10	70 Cal
LUNCH		
Ham (2 oz) with mustard on 2 slices rye bread	300	
Pickle spear	0	
Fresh fruit in season (pear, plum, etc)	70	
Hot or iced tea	10	380 Cal
SNACK		
Handful unsalted mixed nuts	100	
Coffee or tea	10	110 Cal
DINNER		
Frozen Entrée (Appendix D - page 176)	230	
"Big-Bowl Salad"	150	
Fresh fruit in season (pear, plum, etc)	70	
Hot or iced tea	10	460 Cal
SNACK		
Skinny Cow Ice Cream Sandwich	160	
Coffee or tea	10	170 Cal
		1505 Cal

No-Cooking Daily Menu 21

BREAKFAST	Calories	Totals
Orange juice (½ cup)	50	
Soft-boiled egg	80	
Whole-grain toast (2 slices)	140	
Coffee	10	280 Cal
SNACK		
Fresh fruit in season (apple, plum, etc)	70	
Coffee or tea	10	80 Cal
LUNCH		
Soup (Appendix B - page 172)	190	
Small whole-grain roll	80	
Nature Valley Crunchy Granola bar	95	
Water	0	365 Cal
SNACK		
Yogurt (4 oz, non-fat any flavor)	60	60 Cal
DINNER		
Frozen Entrée (Appendix D - page 176)	240	
"Big-Bowl Salad"	150	
Whole-grain bread (1 slice)	70	
Fresh fruit in season (apple, peach, plum, etc)	70	
Water with lemon wedge	15	545 Cal
SNACK		
Skinny Cow Ice Cream Sandwich	160	
Coffee or tea	10	170 Cal
		1500 Cal

No-Cooking Daily Menu 22

BREAKFAST	Calories	Totals
Grapefruit (½)	75	
Cheerios (1 cup) + ½ cup skim milk + about 15 raisins	190	
Coffee	10	275 Cal
SNACK		
Handful unsalted mixed nuts	100	
Coffee or tea	10	110 Cal
LUNCH		
Cottage cheese (1 cup low fat)	180	
Fresh fruit in season (apple, peach, etc)	70	
Whole-grain bread (1 slice)	70	
Coffee or tea	10	330 Cal
SNACK		
Kashi TLC Chewy Granola Bar	140	
Coffee or tea	10	150 Cal
DINNER		
Frozen Entrée (Appendix D - page 176)	280	
"Big-Bowl Salad"	150	
Small whole-grain roll	80	
Water	0	510 Cal
SNACK		
Popcorn Mini Bag	110	
Coffee or tea	10	120 Cal
		1495 Cal

No-Cooking Daily Menu 23

BREAKFAST	Calories	Totals
Cantaloupe (½ medium)	50	
Scrambled egg	80	
Toasted whole-grain bread (1 slice)	70	
Coffee	10	210 Cal
SNACK		
Yogurt (4 oz, non-fat any flavor)	60	
Coffee or tea	10	70 Cal
LUNCH		
Soup (Appendix B - page 172)	130	
String cheese (1 piece, any brand)	80	
Fresh fruit in season (apple, plum, etc)	80	
Coffee or tea	10	305 Cal
SNACK		
Handful unsalted mixed nuts	100	
Coffee or tea	10	110 Cal
DINNER		
Frozen Entrée (Appendix D - page 176)	310	
"Big-Bowl Salad"	150	
Whole-grain bread (1 slice)	70	
Fresh fruit in season (apple, plum, etc)	70	
Water with lemon wedge	15	615 Cal
SNACK		
Kashi TLC Crunchy Granola Bar	180	
Coffee or tea	10	190 Cal
		1500 Cal

<h1 style="text-align:center"><u>No-Cooking Daily Menu 24</u></h1>

BREAKFAST	Calories	Totals
Cantaloupe (½ medium)	50	
Oatmeal (½ cup dry) + ½ cup milk + about 15 raisins	220	
Coffee	10	280 Cal
SNACK		
Yogurt (4 oz, non-fat any flavor)	60	
Coffee or tea	10	70 Cal
LUNCH		
Chorizo Egg & Cheese*	260	
Fresh fruit in season (pear, plum, etc)	70	
Diet soda or water	0	330 Cal
* Hot Pockets (wrap)		
SNACK		
Handful unsalted mixed nuts	100	
Coffee or tea	10	110 Cal
DINNER		
Frozen Entrée (Appendix D - page 176)	260	
"Big-Bowl Salad"	150	
Whole-grain bread (1 slice)	70	
Fresh fruit in season (apple, peach, etc)	70	
Water with lemon wedge	15	565 Cal
SNACK		
Kashi TLC Chewy Granola Bar	140	
Coffee or tea	10	150 Cal
		1505 Cal

BREAKFAST	Calories	Totals
Orange juice (½ cup)	50	
Wheaties (¾ cup) + ½ cup skim milk + ½ banana	190	
Whole-grain toast (1 slice)	70	
Coffee	10	320 Cal
SNACK		
Fresh fruit in season (peach, plum, etc)	70	
Coffee or tea	10	80 Cal
LUNCH		
Soup (Appendix B - page 172)	180	
Laughing Cow Light Cheese (2 wedges)	70	
Small whole-grain roll	80	
Coffee or tea	10	340 Cal
SNACK		
Handful unsalted mixed nuts	100	
Coffee or tea	10	110 Cal
DINNER		
Frozen Entrée (Appendix D - page 176)	230	
"Big-Bowl Salad"	150	
Whole-grain bread (1 slice)	70	
Fresh fruit in season (apple, peach, etc)	70	
Water	0	520 Cal
SNACK		
Popcorn Mini Bag	110	
Coffee or tea	10	120 Cal
		1500 Cal

BREAKFAST	Calories	Totals
Orange juice (½ cup)	50	
Kashi Go Lean Waffles (2)	150	
Morningstar Breakfast Sausage Link	80	
Light Syrup (2 Tbsp)	50	
Coffee	10	340 Cal
SNACK		
Yogurt (4 oz, non-fat any flavor)	60	
Coffee or tea	10	70 Cal
LUNCH		
Subway 6" (Ham, Cheese +veggies)*	260	
Fresh fruit in season (apple, peach, plum, etc)	70	
Diet soda	0	330 Cal
SNACK		
Handful unsalted mixed nuts	100	
Coffee or tea	10	110 Cal
DINNER		
Frozen Entrée (Appendix D - page 176)	190	
"Big-Bowl Salad"	150	
Whole-grain bread (1 slice)	70	
Fresh fruit in season (peach, pear, etc)	70	
Water	0	480 Cal
SNACK		
Skinny Cow Ice Cream Sandwich	160	
Coffee or tea	10	170 Cal
		1500 Cal

No-Cooking Daily Menu 27

BREAKFAST	Calories	Totals
Orange juice (½ cup)	50	
Cheerios (1 cup) + ½ cup skim milk + about 15	190	
Whole grain toast (1 slice)	70	
Coffee	10	320 Cal
SNACK		
Fresh fruit in season (peach, plum, etc)	70	
Coffee or tea	10	80 Cal
LUNCH		
Soup (Appendix B - page 172)	100	
String cheese (1 piece, any brand)	80	
Whole grain bread (1 slice)	70	
Coffee or tea	10	260 Cal
SNACK		
Handful unsalted mixed nuts	100	
Coffee or tea	10	110 Cal
DINNER		
Frozen Entrée (Appendix D - page 176)	300	
"Big-Bowl Salad"	150	
Whole grain bread (1 slice)	70	
Fresh fruit in season (apple, peach, etc)	70	
Water with lemon wedge	15	605 Cal
SNACK		
Popcorn Mini Bag	110	
Coffee or tea	10	120 Cal
		1495 Cal

No-Cooking Daily Menu 28

BREAKFAST	Calories	Totals
Orange juice (½ cup)	50	
Kashi Go Lean Waffles (2)	150	
Morningstar Breakfast Sausage Link	80	
Light Syrup (2 Tbsp)	50	
Coffee	10	340 Cal
SNACK		
Yogurt (4 oz, non-fat any flavor)	60	
Coffee or tea	10	70 Cal
LUNCH		
Ham (2 oz) with mustard on 2 slices rye bread	300	
Laughing Cow Light Cheese (1 wedge)	35	
Fresh fruit in season (apple, peach, etc)	70	
Coffee or tea	10	415 Cal
SNACK		
Handful unsalted mixed nuts	100	
Coffee or tea	10	110 Cal
DINNER		
Frozen Entrée (Appendix D - page 176)	160	
"Big-Bowl Salad"	150	
Whole grain bread (1 slice)	70	
Water with lemon wedge	15	395 Cal
SNACK		
Skinny Cow Ice Cream Sandwich	160	
Coffee or tea	10	170 Cal
		1500 Cal

BREAKFAST	Calories	Totals
Grapefruit (½)	75	
Fried egg (1)	80	
Turkey bacon (1 slice)	35	
Whole grain toast (1 slice)	70	
Coffee	10	270 Cal
SNACK		
Yogurt (4 oz, non-fat any flavor)	60	
Coffee or tea	10	70 Cal
LUNCH		
Soup (Appendix B - page 172)	160	
String cheese (1 piece, any brand)	80	
Fresh fruit in season (apple, peach, etc)	70	
Coffee or tea	10	320 Cal
SNACK		
Handful unsalted mixed nuts	100	
Coffee or tea	10	110 Cal
DINNER		
Frozen Entrée (Appendix D - page 176)	250	
"Big-Bowl Salad"	150	
Whole-grain bread (1 slice)	70	
Fresh fruit in season (apple, peach, etc)	70	
Water	0	540 Cal
SNACK		
Kashi TLC Crunchy Granola Bar	180	
Coffee or tea	10	190 Cal
		1500 Cal

No-Cooking Daily Menu 30

BREAKFAST	Calories	Totals
Grapefruit (½)	75	
Wheaties (¾ cup) + ½ cup skim milk + ½ banana	190	
Coffee	10	275 Cal
SNACK		
Handful unsalted mixed nuts	100	
Coffee or tea	10	110 Cal
LUNCH		
Cottage cheese (1 cup low fat)	180	
Fresh fruit in season (apple, plum, etc)	70	
Small whole-grain roll	80	
Coffee or tea	10	340 Cal
SNACK		
Kashi TLC Crunchy Granola Bar	180	
Coffee or tea	10	190 Cal
DINNER		
Frozen Entrée (Appendix D - page 176)	270	
"Big-Bowl Salad"	150	
Whole-grain bread (1 slice)	70	
Water with lemon wedge	15	500 Cal
SNACK		
Fresh fruit in season (pear, plum, etc)	70	
Coffee or tea	10	80 Cal
		1495 Cal

No-Cooking Daily Menu 31

BREAKFAST	Calories	Totals
Cantaloupe (½ medium)	50	
Perfect egg (Recipe 8a - page 124)	80	
Toasted raisin bread (1 slice)	75	
Coffee	10	215 Cal
SNACK		
Yogurt (4 oz, non-fat any flavor)	60	60 Cal
LUNCH		
Soup (Appendix B - page 172)*	280	
Whole-grain bread (1 slice)	70	
Banana (1 medium)	100	
Water	0	450 Cal
* Enjoy 2 servings of a 140 Calorie soup.		
SNACK		
Fresh fruit in season (peach, plum, etc)	70	
Coffee or tea	10	80 Cal
DINNER		
Frozen Entrée (Appendix D - page 176)	200	
"Big-Bowl Salad"	150	
Small whole-grain roll	80	
Glass of wine (4 oz)	100	
Water	0	530 Cal
SNACK		
Skinny Cow Ice Cream Sandwich	160	
Coffee or tea	10	170 Cal
		1505 Cal

No-Cooking Daily Menu 32

BREAKFAST	Calories	Totals
Tomato juice (½ cup)	20	
Shredded Wheat (1 cup) + ½ cup skim milk + ½ banana	265	
Coffee	10	295 Cal
SNACK		
Yogurt (4 oz, non-fat any flavor)	60	
Coffee or tea	10	70 Cal
LUNCH		
Chicken Broccoli & Cheddar*	270	
Fresh fruit in season (apple, plum, etc)	70	
Diet soda or water	0	340 Cal
* Hot Pockets (wrap).		
SNACK		
Handful unsalted mixed nuts	100	
Coffee or tea	10	110 Cal
DINNER		
Frozen Entrée (Appendix D - page 176)	220	
"Big-Bowl Salad"	150	
Whole-grain bread (1 slice)	70	
Fresh blueberries, cherries or grapes (1 cup)	100	
Water	0	540 Cal
SNACK		
Kashi TLC Chewy Granola Bar	140	
Coffee or tea	10	150 Cal
		1505 Cal

No-Cooking Daily Menu 33

BREAKFAST	Calories	Totals
Orange juice (½ cup)	50	
Wheat Chex (¾ cup) + ½ cup skim milk + ½ banana	250	
Coffee	10	310 Cal
SNACK		
Fresh fruit in season (apple, plum, etc)	70	
Coffee or tea	10	80 Cal
LUNCH		
Soup (Appendix B - page 172)	90	
String cheese (1 piece, any brand)	80	
Whole-grain bread (1 slice)	70	
Coffee or tea	10	250 Cal
SNACK		
Handful unsalted mixed nuts	100	
Coffee or tea	10	110 Cal
DINNER		
Frozen Entrée (Appendix D - page 176)	320	
"Big-Bowl Salad"	150	
Whole-grain bread (1 slice)	70	
Fresh fruit in season (apple, plum, etc)	70	
Water with lemon wedge	15	625 Cal
SNACK		
Popcorn Mini Bag	110	
Coffee or tea	10	120 Cal
		1495 Cal

No-Cooking Daily Menu 34

BREAKFAST	Calories	Totals
Fresh or frozen strawberries (½ cup)	25	
Kashi Go Lean Waffles (2)	150	
Morningstar Breakfast Sausage Link	80	
Light Syrup (2 Tbsp)	50	
Coffee	10	315 Cal
SNACK		
Yogurt (4 oz, non-fat any flavor)	60	
Coffee or tea	10	70 Cal
LUNCH		
Subway 6" (Turkey breast, Cheese +veggies)	230	
Fresh fruit in season (apple, plum, etc)	70	
Diet soda or water	0	300 Cal
SNACK		
Handful unsalted mixed nuts	100	
Coffee or tea	10	110 Cal
DINNER		
Frozen Entrée (Appendix D - page 176)	300	
"Big-Bowl Salad"	150	
Whole-grain bread (1 slice)	70	
Water with lemon wedge	15	535 Cal
SNACK		
Skinny Cow Ice Cream Sandwich	160	
Coffee or tea	10	170 Cal
		1500 Cal

No-Cooking Daily Menu 35

BREAKFAST	Calories	Totals
Grapefruit (½)	75	
Fried egg	80	
Whole grain toast (1 slice)	70	
Coffee	10	235 Cal
SNACK		
Yogurt (4 oz, non-fat any flavor)	60	
Coffee or tea	10	70 Cal
LUNCH		
Salad (3 oz canned tuna, 1 tsp Evoo, onions, celery)	175	
String cheese (1 piece, any brand - 80 Cal max)	80	
Rye bread (1 slice)	70	
Hot or iced tea	10	335 Cal
SNACK		
Handful unsalted mixed nuts	100	
Coffee or tea	10	110 Cal
DINNER		
Frozen Entrée (Appendix D - page 176)	340	
"Big-Bowl Salad"	150	
Whole-grain bread (1 slice)	70	
Fresh fruit in season (peach, plum, etc)	70	
Water	0	630 Cal
SNACK		
Popcorn Mini Bag	110	
Coffee or tea	10	120 Cal
		1500 Cal

BREAKFAST	Calories	Totals
Fresh sliced orange	75	
Cheerios (1 cup) + ½ cup skim milk + about 15 raisins	190	
Whole grain toast (1 slice)	70	
Coffee	10	345 Cal
SNACK		
Handful unsalted mixed nuts	100	
Coffee or tea	10	110 Cal
LUNCH		
Cottage cheese (1 cup low fat)	180	
Fresh fruit in season (pear, plum, etc)	70	
Small whole-grain roll	80	
Coffee or tea	10	340 Cal
SNACK		
Kashi TLC Chewy Granola Bar	140	
Coffee or tea	10	150 Cal
DINNER		
Frozen Entrée (Appendix D - page 176)	220	
"Big-Bowl Salad"	150	
Whole-grain bread (1 slice)	70	
Water	0	440 Cal
SNACK		
Popcorn Mini Bag	110	
Coffee or tea	10	120 Cal
		1505 Cal

No-Cooking Daily Menu 37

BREAKFAST	Calories	Totals
Grapefruit (½)	75	
Soft-boiled egg	80	
Turkey bacon (1 slice)	35	
Whole-grain toast (1 slice)	70	
Coffee	10	270 Cal
SNACK		
Fresh fruit in season (apple, plum, etc)	70	
Coffee or tea	10	80 Cal
LUNCH		
Soup (Appendix B - page 172)	220	
Laughing Cow Light Cheese (1 wedge)	35	
Small whole-grain roll	80	
Hot or iced tea	10	345 Cal
SNACK		
Yogurt (4 oz, non-fat any flavor)	60	
Coffee or tea	10	70 Cal
DINNER		
Frozen Entrée (Appendix D - page 176)	330	
"Big-Bowl Salad"	150	
Fresh fruit in season (apple, plum, etc)	70	
Water with lemon wedge	15	565 Cal
SNACK		
Skinny Cow Ice Cream Sandwich	160	
Coffee or tea	10	170 Cal
		1490 Cal

No-Cooking Daily Menu 38

BREAKFAST	Calories	Totals
Orange juice (½ cup)	50	
Shredded Wheat (1 cup) + ½ cup skim milk + ½ banana	260	
Coffee	10	320 Cal
SNACK		
Fresh fruit in season (pear, plum, etc)	70	70 Cal
LUNCH		
Peanut butter (2 Tbsp) on 2 slices whole-grain bread	340	
Skim milk (8 oz)	90	
Fresh fruit in season (pear, plum, etc)	70	
Water	0	500 Cal
SNACK		
Nature Valley Crunchy Granola bar	95	
Coffee or tea	10	105 Cal
DINNER		
Frozen Entrée (Appendix D - page 176)	180	
"Big-Bowl Salad"	150	
Whole-grain bread (1 slice)	70	
Diet soda	0	400 Cal
SNACK		
100-Calorie Pack Cookies	100	
Coffee or tea	10	110 Cal
		1505 Cal

BREAKFAST	Calories	Totals
Fresh sliced orange	75	
Wheaties (¾ cup) + ½ cup skim milk + ½ banana	190	
Whole grain toast (1 slice)	70	
Coffee	10	345 Cal
SNACK		
Fresh fruit in season (apple, plum, etc)	70	
Coffee or tea	10	80 Cal
LUNCH		
Soup (Appendix B - page 172)	120	
String cheese (1 piece, any brand)	80	
Small whole-grain roll	80	
Coffee or tea	10	280 Cal
SNACK		
Handful unsalted mixed nuts	100	
Coffee or tea	10	110 Cal
DINNER		
Frozen Entrée (Appendix D - page 176)	330	
"Big-Bowl Salad"	150	
Fresh fruit in season (apple, plum, etc)	70	
Water with lemon wedge	15	565 Cal
SNACK		
Popcorn Mini Bag	110	
Coffee or tea	10	120 Cal
		1500 Cal

No-Cooking Daily Menu 40

BREAKFAST	Calories	Totals
Orange juice (½ cup)	50	
Wheat Chex (¾ cup) + ½ cup skim milk + ½ banana	250	
Coffee	10	310 Cal
SNACK		
Yogurt (4 oz, non-fat any flavor)	60	
Coffee or tea	10	70 Cal
LUNCH		
Ham & Cheddar*	270	
Fresh fruit in season (apple, plum, etc)	70	
Diet soda or water	0	340 Cal
* Hot Pockets Wrap		
SNACK		
Handful unsalted mixed nuts	100	
Coffee or tea	10	110 Cal
DINNER		
Frozen Entrée (Appendix D - page 176)	200	
"Big-Bowl Salad"	150	
Whole-grain bread (1 slice)	70	
Fresh fruit in season (pear, plum, etc)	70	
Water with lemon wedge	15	505 Cal
SNACK		
Skinny Cow Ice Cream Sandwich	160	
Coffee or tea	10	170 Cal
		1505 Cal

No-Cooking Daily Menu 41

BREAKFAST	Calories	Totals
Cantaloupe (½ medium)	50	
Fried egg	80	
Turkey bacon (2 slices)	70	
Toasted raisin bread (1 slice)	75	
Coffee	10	285 Cal
SNACK		
Yogurt (4 oz, non-fat any flavor)	60	
Coffee or tea	10	70 Cal
LUNCH		
Soup (Appendix B - page 172)	170	
String cheese (1 piece, any brand)	80	
Nature Valley Crunchy Granola bar	95	
Coffee or tea	10	355 Cal
SNACK		
Handful unsalted mixed nuts	100	
Coffee or tea	10	110 Cal
DINNER		
Frozen Entrée (Appendix D - page 176)	260	
"Big-Bowl Salad"	150	
Whole-grain bread (1 slice)	70	
Fresh fruit in season (apple, peach, etc)	70	
Hot or iced tea	10	560 Cal
SNACK		
Popcorn Mini Bag	110	
Coffee or tea	10	120 Cal
		1500 Cal

No-Cooking Daily Menu 42

BREAKFAST	Calories	Totals
Grapefruit (½)	75	
Cheerios (1 cup) + ½ cup skim milk + about 15 raisins	190	
Coffee	10	275 Cal
SNACK		
Handful unsalted mixed nuts	100	
Coffee or tea	10	110 Cal
LUNCH		
Cottage cheese (1 cup low fat)	180	
Fresh fruit in season (apple, peach, etc)	70	
Small whole-grain roll	80	
Coffee or tea	10	340 Cal
SNACK		
Kashi TLC Chewy Granola Bar	140	
Coffee or tea	10	150 Cal
DINNER		
Frozen Entrée (Appendix D - page 176)	220	
"Big-Bowl Salad"	150	
Whole-grain bread (1 slice)	70	
Fresh fruit in season (peach, plum, etc)	70	
Water	0	510 Cal
SNACK		
Popcorn Mini Bag	110	
Coffee or tea	10	120 Cal
		1505 Cal

No-Cooking Daily Menu 43

BREAKFAST	Calories	Totals
Grapefruit (½)	75	
Scrambled egg	80	
Whole-grain toast (1 slice)	70	
Coffee	10	235 Cal
SNACK		
Yogurt (4 oz, non-fat any flavor)	60	
Coffee or tea	10	70 Cal
LUNCH		
Soup (Appendix B - page 172)	180	
String cheese (1 piece, any brand)	80	
Small whole-grain roll	80	
Water	0	340 Cal
SNACK		
Handful unsalted mixed nuts	100	
Coffee or tea	10	110 Cal
DINNER		
Frozen Entrée (Appendix D - page 176)	270	
"Big-Bowl Salad"	150	
Whole-grain bread (1 slice)	70	
Fresh fruit in season (apple, pear, etc)	70	
Water with lemon wedge	15	575 Cal
SNACK		
Skinny Cow Ice Cream Sandwich	160	
Coffee or tea	10	170 Cal
		1500 Cal

No-Cooking Daily Menu 44

BREAKFAST	Calories	Totals
Tomato juice (½ cup)	20	
Shredded Wheat (1 cup) + ½ cup skim milk + ½ banana	260	
Coffee	10	290 Cal
SNACK		
Yogurt (4 oz, non-fat any flavor)	60	
Coffee or tea	10	70 Cal
LUNCH		
Ham & Cheddar*	270	
Fresh fruit in season (apple, peach, etc)	70	
Diet soda	0	340 Cal
* Hot Pockets (wrap)		
SNACK		
Handful unsalted mixed nuts	100	
Coffee or tea	10	110 Cal
DINNER		
Frozen Entrée (Appendix D - page 176)	260	
"Big-Bowl Salad"	150	
Whole-grain bread (1 slice)	70	
Fresh fruit in season (peach, plum, etc)	70	
Water	0	550 Cal
SNACK		
Kashi TLC Chewy Granola Bar	140	140 Cal
		1500 Cal

No-Cooking Daily Menu 45

BREAKFAST	Calories	Totals
Cantaloupe (½ medium)	50	
Wheat Chex (¾ cup) + ½ cup skim milk + ½ banana	250	
Coffee	10	310 Cal
SNACK		
Fresh fruit in season (peach, plum, etc)	70	
Coffee or tea	10	80 Cal
LUNCH		
Soup (Appendix B - page 172)	140	
String cheese (1 piece, any brand)	80	
Small whole-grain roll	80	
Coffee or tea	10	310 Cal
SNACK		
Handful unsalted mixed nuts	100	
Coffee or tea	10	110 Cal
DINNER		
Frozen Entrée (Appendix D - page 176)	270	
"Big-Bowl Salad"	150	
Whole-grain bread (1 slice)	70	
Fresh fruit in season (peach, plum, etc)	70	
Fresh fruit in season (peach, plum, etc)	70	570 Cal
SNACK		
Popcorn Mini Bag	110	
Coffee or tea	10	120 Cal
		1500 Cal

Cooking
Daily Meal Plans

Cooking Daily Menu 1

BREAKFAST	Calories	Totals
Grapefruit (½)	75	
Scrambled egg (See **Notes** - page 21)	80	
Turkey Bacon - 2 slices (See **Notes**)	70	
Whole-grain toast (1 slice) (See page 21)	70	
Coffee (See Notes)	10	305 Cal
SNACK		
Yogurt (4 oz, non-fat any flavor)*	60	
Coffee or tea	10	70 Cal
* Such as Dannon Lite & Fit. (Buy 32 oz - use 4 oz.)		
LUNCH		
Ham (2 oz) with mustard on 2 slices rye bread	290	
Pickle spear	0	
Small bunch of grapes	65	
Gelatin dessert (unsweetened)	10	
Hot or iced tea	10	375 Cal
SNACK		
Fresh fruit in season (apple, peach, etc)	70	
Coffee or tea	10	80 Cal
DINNER		
Chicken w Peppers & Onions (Recipe 1 - page 117)	250	
Sautéed red peppers with onions (Recipe 1)	70	
Green beans - steamed & Mashed cauliflower	55	
Large tossed salad with 1½ Tbsp low-cal dressing*	85	
Whole-grain bread (1 slice)	70	
Water with lemon wedge	15	540 Cal
* See page 12.		
SNACK		
Popcorn Mini Bag**	110	
Coffee or tea	10	120 Cal
** Such as Orville Redenbacher's Smart Pop.		1490 Cal

Cooking Daily Menu 2

BREAKFAST	Calories	Totals
Orange juice (½ cup)	50	
Wheaties (¾ cup) + ½ cup skim milk + ½ banana	190	
Coffee	10	250 Cal
SNACK		
Fresh fruit in season (apple, pear, etc)	70	
Coffee or tea	10	80 Cal
LUNCH		
Soup (Appendix B - page 172)	120	
Turkey breast (1 oz) on 1 slice rye bread (½	105	
Pickle spear	0	
Lettuce & tomato slices	20	
Hot or iced tea	10	255 Cal
SNACK		
Popcorn Mini Bag	110	
Coffee or tea	10	120 Cal
DINNER		
Baked Herb-Crusted Cod (Recipe 2 - page 118)	230	
Spinach (½ cup) steamed with garlic & drizzled	100	
Asparagus (7 spear cooked & drained)	20	
Baked potato (medium size) (No Butter!)	100	
Whole grain bread (1 slice)	70	
Fresh fruit in season (apple, plum, etc)	70	
Water with lemon wedge	15	605 Cal
SNACK		
Graham crackers (4 squares)	120	
Skim milk (6 oz)	70	190 Cal
		1500 Cal

Cooking Daily Menu 3

BREAKFAST	Calories	Totals
Fresh or frozen strawberries (½ cup)	25	
French toasted English Muffin (Recipe 3 - page 119)	270	
Light syrup (1 Tbsp)	30	
Coffee	10	335 Cal
SNACK		
Handful unsalted mixed nuts	100	100 Cal
LUNCH		
Salad (3 oz canned tuna, 1 tsp Evoo, onions, celery)	175	
Lettuce & tomato wedges	20	
Rye bread (1 slice)	70	
Fresh fruit in season (apple, peach, etc)	70	
Coffee or tea	10	345 Cal
SNACK		
Popcorn Mini Bag	110	
Coffee or tea	10	120 Cal
DINNER		
Broiled veal chop (4 oz lean)	200	
Corn on the cob (1 medium ear) (No Butter!)	100	
Broccoli (½ cup steamed & drizzled with 1 tsp	70	
Large tossed salad with 1½ Tbsp low-cal dressing	85	
Water	0	455 Cal
SNACK		
100-Calorie Pack Cookies*	100	
Skim milk (4 oz)	45	145 Cal
* Such as Nabisco Oreo/Chips Ahoy/etc.		1500 Cal

<u>Cooking Daily Menu 4</u>

BREAKFAST	Calories	Totals
Grapefruit (½)	75	
Cheerios (1 cup) + ½ cup skim milk + about 15 raisins*	190	
Coffee	10	275 Cal
SNACK		
Fresh fruit in season (apple, plum, etc)	70	
Coffee or tea	10	80 Cal
LUNCH		
Cottage cheese (1 cup low fat)	180	
Tossed salad with 2 Tbsp low-cal dressing	85	
Small whole-grain roll	80	
Hot or iced tea	10	355 Cal
SNACK		
Handful unsalted mixed nuts	100	100 Cal
DINNER		
Meat Loaf (Recipe 4 - page 120)	290	
One-half acorn squash (baked with ½ tsp maple	90	
Spinach (½ cup steamed & drizzled with 1 tsp	70	
Romaine lettuce, tomato slices & 1 Tbsp low-cal	45	
Gelatin dessert (unsweetened)	10	
Water with lemon wedge	15	520 Cal
SNACK		
Two small cookies	160	
Coffee or tea	10	170 Cal
*** See Notes** page 13 re substituting blueberries for raisins.		1500 Cal

Cooking Daily Menu 5

BREAKFAST	Calories	Totals
Fresh orange sliced	75	
Kashi Go Lean cereal (1 cup) + ½ cup skim milk	185	
Coffee	10	270 Cal
SNACK		
Handful unsalted mixed nuts	100	
Coffee or tea	10	110 Cal
LUNCH		
Subway 6" (Turkey breast, Cheese +veggies)*	230	
Diet soda or water	0	230 Cal
* Half whole-grain roll		
SNACK		
Dark chocolate (1 oz)	150	
Coffee or tea	10	160 Cal
DINNER		
Veal w Mushrooms & Tomato (Recipe 5 - page 121)	520	
Small whole-grain roll	80	
Hot or iced tea	10	610 Cal
SNACK		
Popcorn Mini Bag	110	
Coffee or tea	10	120 Cal
		1500 Cal

Cooking Daily Menu 6

BREAKFAST	Calories	Totals
Tomato juice (½ cup)	20	
Shredded Wheat (1 cup) + ½ cup skim milk + ½ banana	265	
Coffee	10	**295 Cal**
SNACK		
Handful unsalted mixed nuts	100	
Coffee or tea	10	**110 Cal**
LUNCH		
Leftover meat loaf (½ Day 4 serving) with ketchup	155	
Small whole-grain roll	80	
Lettuce	0	
Fresh or frozen berries (½ cup)	50	
Water with lemon wedge	15	**300 Cal**
SNACK		
Yogurt (4 oz nonfat, any flavor)	60	
Coffee or tea	10	**70 Cal**
DINNER		
Pizza (Recipe 6 - page 122)	350	
Large tossed salad with 1½ Tbsp low-cal dressing	70	
Fresh fruit in season (apple, peach, etc)	70	
Glass of red wine (4 oz)	100	
Water with lemon wedge	15	**605 Cal**
SNACK		
100-Calorie Pack Cookies	100	
Coffee or tea	10	**110 Cal**
		1490 Cal

Cooking Daily Menu 7

BREAKFAST	Calories	Totals
Cantaloupe (½ medium)	50	
Oatmeal (½ cup dry) + ½ cup skim milk + about 15 raisins	220	
Coffee	10	280 Cal
SNACK		
Handful unsalted mixed nuts	100	
Coffee or tea	10	110 Cal
LUNCH		
Soup (Appendix B - page 172)	140	
Grilled cheese sandwich (2 slices 2% cheese)	240	
Lettuce and sliced tomato	20	
Pickle spear	0	
Hot or iced tea	0	360 Cal
SNACK		
Popcorn Mini Bag	110	
Coffee or tea	10	120 Cal
DINNER		
Baked salmon with salsa (Recipe 7 - page 123)	215	
Baked summer squash and zucchini	40	
Brown rice (½ cup – after cooking)	100	
Large tossed salad with 1½ Tbsp low-cal dressing	85	
Whole-grain bread (1 slice)	70	
Water with lemon wedge	15	525 Cal
SNACK		
100-Calorie Pack Cookies	100	
Coffee or tea	10	110 Cal
		1505 Cal

Cooking Daily Menu 8

BREAKFAST	Calories	Totals
Orange juice (½ cup)	50	
Perfect egg (Recipe 8a - page 124)	80	
Whole-grain toast (2 slices)	140	
Coffee	10	280 Cal
SNACK		
Yogurt (4 oz nonfat, any flavor)	60	
Coffee or tea	10	70 Cal
LUNCH		
Salad (3 oz canned tuna, 1 tsp Evoo, onions, celery)	175	
Lettuce & tomato wedges + rye bread (1 slice)	60	
Fresh fruit in season (apple, plum, etc)	70	
Hot or iced tea	10	315 Cal
SNACK		
Handful unsalted mixed nuts	100	
Coffee or tea	10	110 Cal
DINNER		
Veggie burger – (1 patty) (Recipe 8b - page 125)	100	
Low-fat cheddar cheese (1 thin slice)	50	
Seeded hamburger roll	140	
Beets (3 small, boiled, skinned & sliced)	45	
Large tossed salad with 1½ Tbsp low-cal dressing	85	
Fresh fruit in season (apple, peach, etc)	70	
Water with lemon wedge	15	505 Cal
SNACK		
Graham crackers (5 squares)	150	
Skim milk (6 oz)	70	210 Cal
		1500 Cal

Cooking Daily Menu 9

BREAKFAST	Calories	Totals
Orange juice (½ cup)	50	
Wild blueberry pancakes (Recipe 9 - page 126)	190	
Turkey bacon (2 slices)	70	
Light syrup (1½ Tbsp)	45	
Coffee	10	365 Cal
SNACK		
Yogurt (4 oz nonfat, any flavor)	60	
Coffee or tea	10	70 Cal
LUNCH		
Peanut butter (2 Tbsp) on 2 slices whole-grain bread	340	
Skim milk (6 oz)	65	
Fresh fruit in season (apple, plum, etc)	70	475 Cal
SNACK		
Handful unsalted mixed nuts	100	
Coffee or tea	10	110 Cal
DINNER		
Broiled pork chop (about 4 oz of meat - trimmed of fat)	260	
Green peas (½ cup)	55	
Tomato & cucumber salad with 1½ Tbsp low-cal	70	
Water	0	385 Cal
SNACK		
Fiber One Chocolate Fudge Brownie	90	
Coffee or tea	10	100 Cal
		1505 Cal

<h1 align="center"><u>Cooking Daily Menu 10</u></h1>

<u>BREAKFAST</u>	<u>Calories</u>	<u>Totals</u>
Fresh sliced orange	**75**	
Cheerios (1 cup) + ½ cup skim milk + about 15 raisins	**190**	
Whole-grain toast (1 slice)	**70**	
Coffee	**10**	**345 Cal**
<u>SNACK</u>		
Handful unsalted mixed nuts	**100**	
Coffee or tea	**10**	**110 Cal**
<u>LUNCH</u>		
Cottage cheese (1 cup low fat)	**180**	
Large tossed salad with 1½ Tbsp low-cal dressing	**85**	
Small whole-grain roll	**80**	
Water	**0**	**345 Cal**
<u>SNACK</u>		
Fresh fruit in season (apple, plum, etc)	**70**	
Coffee or tea	**10**	**80 Cal**
<u>DINNER</u>		
Grilled chicken sausage (2 links - 2½ oz per link)	**180**	
Artichoke-bean salad (Recipe 10 - page 127)	**190**	
Green beans (¼ lb – steamed)	**25**	
Whole-grain bread (1 slice)	**70**	
Water	**0**	**465 Cal**
<u>SNACK</u>		
Skinny Cow Ice Cream Sandwich	**160**	**160 Cal**
		1505 Cal

Cooking Daily Menu 11

BREAKFAST	Calories	Totals
Orange juice (½ cup)	50	
Shredded Wheat (1 cup) + ½ cup skim milk + ½ banana	260	
Whole-grain toast (1 slice)	70	
Coffee	10	390 Cal
SNACK		
Popcorn Mini Bag	110	
Coffee or tea	10	120 Cal
LUNCH		
Turkey frank (2 oz) with mustard & relish	150	
Hot-dog bun	130	
Hot or iced tea	10	290 Cal
SNACK		
Yogurt (4 oz nonfat, any flavor)	60	
Coffee or tea	10	70 Cal
DINNER		
Pasta with Marinara sauce (Recipe 11 - page 128)	225	
Large tossed salad with 1½ Tbsp low-cal dressing	85	
Fresh fruit in season (peach, plum, etc)	70	
Italian or French bread (1 slice)	80	
Water with lemon wedge	15	475 Cal
SNACK		
Kashi TLC Chewy Granola Bar	140	
Coffee or tea	10	150 Cal
		1495 Cal

Cooking Daily Menu 12

BREAKFAST	Calories	Totals
Fresh or frozen strawberries (1 cup)	50	
French toasted English Muffin (Recipe 3 - page 110)	270	
Light syrup (1½ Tbsp)	45	
Coffee	10	375 Cal
SNACK		
Yogurt (4 oz nonfat, any flavor)	60	
Coffee or tea	10	70 Cal
LUNCH		
Salad (3 oz canned tuna, 1 tsp Evoo, onions, celery)	175	
Lettuce & tomato wedges	20	
Rye bread (1 slice)	70	
Coffee or tea	10	275 Cal
SNACK		
Handful unsalted mixed nuts	100	
Coffee or tea	10	110 Cal
DINNER		
London broil (Recipe 12 - page 129)	320	
Brown rice (½ cup – after cooking)	100	
Steamed broccoli (1 cup – after cooking)	50	
Fresh fruit in season (apple, plum, etc)	70	
Water with lemon wedge	15	555 Cal
SNACK		
100-Calorie Pack Cookies	100	
Coffee or tea	10	110 Cal
		1495 Cal

Cooking Daily Menu 13

BREAKFAST	Calories	Totals
Orange juice (½ cup)	50	
Kashi GoLean (1 cup) + ½ cup skim milk + ½ banana	235	
Whole-grain toast (1 slice)	70	
Coffee	10	365 Cal
SNACK		
Fresh fruit in season (apple, plum, etc)	70	
Coffee or tea	10	80 Cal
LUNCH		
Soup (Appendix B - page 172)	100	
Small whole-grain roll	80	
Lettuce & tomato with 1 Tbsp low-cal dressing	45	
Laughing Cow Light Cheese (2 wedges)	70	
Hot or iced tea	10	305 Cal
SNACK		
Graham crackers (4 squares)	120	
Coffee or tea	10	130 Cal
DINNER		
Baked red snapper (Recipe 13 - page 130)	215	
Wild rice mix (Recipe 13)	160	
Green beans & tomato	75	
Water	0	450 Cal
SNACK		
Skinny Cow Ice Cream Sandwich	160	
Coffee or tea	10	170 Cal
		1500 Cal

Cooking Daily Menu 14

BREAKFAST	Calories	Totals
Cantaloupe (½ medium)	50	
Ideal egg (Recipe 8a - page 115)	80	
Turkey bacon (2 slices)	70	
Toasted raisin bread (1 slice)	75	
Coffee	10	285 Cal
SNACK		
Yogurt (4 oz nonfat, any flavor)	60	
Coffee or tea	10	70 Cal
LUNCH		
Ham & Cheddar*	270	
Fresh fruit in season (pear, plum, etc)	70	
Cucumber slices and carrots and celery sticks	15	
Hot or iced tea	10	365 Cal
* Hot Pockets Wrap		
SNACK		
Handful unsalted mixed nuts	100	
Coffee or tea	10	110 Cal
DINNER		
Cajun chicken salad (Recipe 14 - page 131)	330	
Whole-grain bread (1 slice)	70	
Hot or iced tea	10	
Fresh fruit in season (apple, plum, etc)	70	480 Cal
SNACK		
Kashi TLC Crunchy Granola Bar	180	
Coffee or tea	10	190 Cal
		1500 Cal

Cooking Daily Menu 15

BREAKFAST	Calories	Totals
Grapefruit (½)	75	
Cheerios (1 cup) + ½ cup skim milk + about 15 raisins	190	
Coffee	10	275 Cal
SNACK		
Handful unsalted mixed nuts	100	
Coffee or tea	10	110 Cal
LUNCH		
Cottage cheese (1 cup low fat)	180	
Large tossed salad with 1½ Tbsp low-cal dressing	70	
Small whole-grain roll	80	
Water with lemon wedge	15	345 Cal
SNACK		
Fresh fruit in season (peach, plum, etc)	70	
Coffee or tea	10	80 Cal
DINNER		
Grilled swordfish (Recipe 15 - page 132)	250	
Grilled potatoes (Day 15 Recipe)	100	
Grilled cherry tomatoes (Day 15 Recipe)	45	
Spinach (½ cup) steamed with garlic & drizzled	50	
Whole-grain bread (1 slice)	70	
Water with lemon wedge	15	530 Cal
SNACK		
Kashi TLC Chewy Granola Bar	140	
Coffee or tea	10	150 Cal
		1490 Cal

Cooking Daily Menu 16

BREAKFAST	Calories	Totals
Tomato juice (¾ cup)	30	
Shredded Wheat (1 cup) + ½ cup skim milk + ½ banana	260	
Coffee	10	300 Cal
SNACK		
Handful unsalted mixed nuts	100	
Coffee or tea	10	110 Cal
LUNCH		
Ham (2 oz) with mustard on 2 slices rye bread	290	
Pickle spear	0	
Hot or iced tea	10	300 Cal
SNACK		
Yogurt (4 oz nonfat, any flavor)	60	
Coffee or tea	10	70 Cal
DINNER		
Spaghetti alla Puttanesca (Recipe 16 - page 133)	345	
Large tossed salad with 1½ Tbsp low-cal dressing	85	
Italian or French bread (1 slice)	80	
Glass of red wine (4 oz)	100	
Hot or iced tea	10	610 Cal
SNACK		
100-Calorie Pack Cookies	100	
Coffee or tea	10	110 Cal
		1500 Cal

Cooking Daily Menu 17

BREAKFAST	Calories	Totals
Fresh or frozen strawberries (1 cup)	25	
French toasted English Muffin (Recipe 3 - page 119)	270	
Light syrup (1 Tbsp)	30	
Coffee	10	335 Cal
SNACK		
Yogurt (4 oz nonfat, any flavor)	60	
Coffee or tea	10	70 Cal
LUNCH		
Soup (Appendix B - page 172)	100	
BLT sandwich (2 slices turkey bacon, 1 Tbsp light mayo)	245	
Pickle spear	0	
Hot or iced tea	10	355 Cal
SNACK		
Popcorn Mini Bag	110	
Coffee or tea	10	120 Cal
DINNER		
Shrimp & spinach salad (Recipe 17 - page 134)	310	
Whole-grain bread (1 slice)	70	
Fresh fruit in season (apple, peach, etc)	70	
Water	0	450 Cal
SNACK		
Skinny Cow Ice Cream Sandwich	160	
Coffee or tea	10	170 Cal
		1500 Cal

Cooking Daily Menu 18

BREAKFAST	Calories	Totals
Grapefruit (½)	75	
Cheerios (1 cup) + ½ cup skim milk + about 15 raisins	190	
Coffee	10	275 Cal
SNACK		
Fresh fruit in season (pear, plum, etc)	70	70 Cal
LUNCH		
Cottage cheese (1 cup low fat)	180	
Large tossed salad with 1½ Tbsp low-cal dressing	85	
Small whole-grain roll	80	
Hot or iced tea	10	355 Cal
SNACK		
Handful unsalted mixed nuts	100	100 Cal
DINNER		
Hanger steak (Recipe 18 - page 135)	320	
Roasted potatoes (Recipe 18)	120	
Cherry tomatoes (Recipe 18)	20	
Steamed spinach (½ cup)	25	
Whole-grain bread (1 slice)	70	
Water	0	555 Cal
SNACK		
Kashi TLC Chewy Granola Bar	140	
Coffee or tea	10	150 Cal
		1505 Cal

Cooking Daily Menu 19

BREAKFAST	Calories	Totals
Fresh orange sliced	75	
Soft-boiled egg	80	
Whole-grain toast (2 slices)	70	
Coffee	10	305 Cal
SNACK		
Yogurt (4 oz nonfat, any flavor)	60	60 Cal
LUNCH		
Salad – 3 oz canned salmon, 1 tsp Evoo, onions & celery	200	
Lettuce & tomato wedges	20	
Rye bread (1 slice)	70	
Fresh fruit in season (apple, peach, etc)	70	
Coffee or tea	10	370 Cal
SNACK		
Handful unsalted mixed nuts	100	
Coffee or tea	10	110 Cal
DINNER		
Chicken breast (5 oz - broiled)	250	
Four bean plus salad (½ cup) (Recipe 19 - page 136)	135	
Large tossed salad with 1½ Tbsp low-cal dressing	85	
Water with lemon wedge	15	485 Cal
SNACK		
Skinny Cow Ice Cream Sandwich	160	
Coffee or tea	10	170 Cal
		1500 Cal

Cooking Daily Menu 20

BREAKFAST	Calories	Totals
Cantaloupe (½ medium)	50	
Wheaties (¾ cup) + ½ cup skim milk + ½ banana	190	
Whole-grain toast (1 slice)	70	
Coffee	10	320 Cal
SNACK		
Handful unsalted mixed nuts	100	
Coffee or tea	10	110 Cal
LUNCH		
Ham (2 oz) with mustard on 2 slices rye bread	300	
Pickle spear	0	
Small bunch of grapes	65	
Hot or iced tea	10	375 Cal
SNACK		
Yogurt (4 oz nonfat, any flavor)	60	
Coffee or tea	10	70 Cal
DINNER		
Beans & Greens Salad (Recipe 20 - page 137)	260	
Whole-grain bread (1 slice)	70	
Baked potato (medium)	100	
Fresh fruit in season (apple, plum, etc)	70	
Water with lemon wedge	15	515 Cal
SNACK		
100-Calorie Pack Cookies	100	
Coffee or tea	10	110 Cal
		1500 Cal

Cooking Daily Menu 21

BREAKFAST	Calories	Totals
Cantaloupe (½ medium)	50	
Fried eggs (2 eggs)	160	
Toasted whole-grain bread (1 slice)	70	
Coffee	10	290 Cal
SNACK		
Fresh fruit in season (apple, peach, etc)	70	
Coffee or tea	10	80 Cal
LUNCH		
Soup (Appendix B - page 172)	160	
Hard whole-grain roll (medium)	80	
Lettuce & tomato slices	20	
Small bunch of grapes	65	
Hot or iced tea	10	335 Cal
SNACK		
Handful unsalted mixed nuts	100	
Coffee or tea	10	110 Cal
DINNER		
Grilled scallops (Recipe 21 - page 138)	210	
Grilled polenta (Recipe 21)	125	
Mushroom-steamed green beans-red onion	45	
Grilled asparagus	10	
Large tossed salad with 1½ Tbsp low-cal dressing	85	
Water	0	475 Cal
SNACK		
Graham crackers (4 squares)	120	
Skim milk (8 oz)	90	210 Cal
		1500 Cal

Cooking Daily Menu 22

BREAKFAST	Calories	Totals
Orange juice (½ cup)	50	
Oatmeal (½ cup dry) + ½ cup skim milk + about 15 raisins	220	
Coffee	10	280 Cal
SNACK		
Fresh fruit in season (apple, plum, etc)	70	
Coffee or tea	10	80 Cal
LUNCH		
One serving left over Day 20 bean salad	260	
Small whole-grain roll	80	
Lettuce & tomato slices	20	
Hot or iced tea	10	370 Cal
SNACK		
Yogurt (4 oz nonfat, any flavor)	60	
Coffee or tea	10	70 Cal
DINNER		
Fettuccine (Recipe 22 - page 139)	290	
Large tossed salad with 1½ Tbsp low-cal dressing	85	
Italian or French bread (1 slice)	80	
Glass of red wine (4 oz)	100	
Water	0	555 Cal
SNACK		
Kashi TLC Chewy Granola Bar	140	
Coffee or tea	10	150 Cal
		1505 Cal

Cooking Daily Menu 23

BREAKFAST	Calories	Totals
Fresh sliced orange	75	
Wild blueberry pancakes (Recipe 9 - page 126)	190	
Turkey bacon (2 slices)	70	
Light syrup (2 Tbsp)	60	
Coffee	10	405 Cal
SNACK		
Yogurt (4 oz nonfat, any flavor)	60	
Coffee or tea	10	70 Cal
LUNCH		
Salad (3 oz canned tuna, 1 tsp Evoo, onions, celery)	175	
Lettuce & tomato wedges	20	
Rye bread (1 slice)	70	
Fresh fruit in season (apple, peach, etc)	70	
Water with lemon wedge	15	350 Cal
SNACK		
Handful unsalted mixed nuts	100	
Coffee or tea	10	110 Cal
DINNER		
Barbequed shrimp (Recipe 23 - page 140)	160	
Corn on the cob (medium)	60	
Steamed broccoli (1 cup – after cooking)	50	
Small whole-grain roll	80	
Water with lemon wedge	15	365 Cal
SNACK		
Graham crackers (4 squares)	120	
Skim milk (6 oz)	70	190 Cal
		1490 Cal

Cooking Daily Menu 24

BREAKFAST	Calories	Totals
Fresh orange sliced	75	
Kashi GoLean (1 cup) + ½ cup skim milk + ½ banana	235	
Coffee	10	320 Cal
SNACK		
Fresh fruit in season (apple, plum, etc)	70	
Coffee or tea	10	80 Cal
LUNCH		
Subway 6" (Turkey breast, Cheese +veggies)*	230	
Small bunch of grapes	50	
Diet soda or water	0	280 Cal
SNACK		
Graham crackers (4 squares)	120	
Coffee or tea	10	130 Cal
DINNER		
Cheeseburger (Recipe 24 - page 141)	370	
Lettuce and sliced tomato	20	
Whole-grain hard roll	140	
Steamed green beans	25	
Pickle spear	0	
Water with lemon wedge	15	570 Cal
SNACK		
Popcorn Mini Bag	110	
Coffee or tea	10	120 Cal
		1500 Cal

Cooking Daily Menu 25

BREAKFAST	Calories	Totals
Grapefruit (½)	75	
Scrambled egg	80	
Turkey bacon - 2 slices	70	
Whole-grain toast (1 slice)	70	
Coffee	10	305 Cal
SNACK		
Yogurt (4 oz nonfat, any flavor)	60	60 Cal
LUNCH		
Ham (2 oz) with mustard on 2 slices rye bread	300	
Pickle spear	0	
Small bunch of grapes	65	
Hot or iced tea	10	375 Cal
SNACK		
Fresh fruit in season (apple, plum, etc)	70	
Coffee or tea	10	80 Cal
DINNER		
Baked Sea Bass (Recipe 25 - page 142)	395	
Large tossed salad with 1½ Tbsp low-cal dressing	85	
Water with lemon wedge	15	495 Cal
SNACK		
Kashi TLC Chewy Granola Bar	140	
Skim milk (4 oz)	45	185 Cal
		1500 Cal

Cooking Daily Menu 26

BREAKFAST	Calories	Totals
Grapefruit (½)	75	
Cheerios (1 cup) + ½ cup skim milk + about 15 raisins	190	
Coffee	10	275 Cal
SNACK		
Fresh fruit in season (pear, plum, etc)	70	70 Cal
LUNCH		
Cottage cheese (1 cup low fat)	180	
Tossed salad with 1½ Tbsp low-cal dressing	85	
Small whole-grain roll	80	
Water	0	345 Cal
SNACK		
Handful unsalted mixed nuts	100	
Coffee or tea	10	110 Cal
DINNER		
Turkey tenders & veggies (Recipe 26 - page 143)	350	
Spinach (½ cup steamed & drizzled with 1 tsp	70	
Romaine lettuce, tomato slices & 1 Tbsp low-cal	45	
Whole-grain bread (1 slice)	70	
Water	0	535 Cal
SNACK		
Two small cookies	160	
Coffee or tea	10	170 Cal
		1505 Cal

Cooking Daily Menu 27

BREAKFAST	Calories	Totals
Tomato juice (½ cup)	20	
Shredded Wheat (1 cup) + ½ cup skim milk + ½ banana	265	
Coffee	10	295 Cal
SNACK		
Handful unsalted mixed nuts	100	
Coffee or tea	10	110 Cal
LUNCH		
Roast beef (2 oz) with lettuce sandwich	300	
Hot or iced tea	10	310 Cal
SNACK		
Fresh fruit in season (pear, plum, etc)	70	
Coffee or tea	10	80 Cal
DINNER		
Pasta Rapini (Recipe 27 - page 144)	290	
Large tossed green salad with 1½ Tbsp low-cal	85	
Fresh fruit in season (apple, peach, etc)	85	
Italian or French bread (1 slice)	80	
Glass of red wine (4 oz)	100	
Water	0	640 Cal
SNACK		
Graham Crackers (2 squares)	60	
Coffee or tea	10	70 Cal
		1505 Cal

Cooking Daily Menu 28

BREAKFAST	Calories	Totals
Cantaloupe (½ medium)	50	
Wheaties (¾ cup) + ½ cup skim milk + ½ banana	190	
Whole grain toast (1 slice)	70	
Coffee	10	320 Cal
SNACK		
Fresh fruit in season (apple, pear, etc)	70	
Coffee or tea	10	80 Cal
LUNCH		
Soup (Appendix B - page 172)	130	
Turkey (1 oz) on 1 slice of rye bread (½ sandwich)	120	
Lettuce & tomato slices	20	
Hot or iced tea	10	280 Cal
SNACK		
Kashi TLC Chewy Granola Bar	140	
Coffee or tea	10	150 Cal
DINNER		
Grilled Tilapia (Recipe 28 - page 145)	300	
Asparagus spears(6)	25	
Wild rice (½ cup – after cooking)	100	
Large tossed salad with 1½ Tbsp low-cal dressing	85	
Water	0	510 Cal
SNACK		
Graham crackers (3 squares)	90	
Skim milk (6 oz)	70	160 Cal
		1500 Cal

Cooking Daily Menu 29

BREAKFAST	Calories	Totals
Orange juice (½ cup)	50	
Soft-boiled egg	80	
Whole grain toast (2 slices)	140	
Coffee	10	280 Cal
SNACK		
Yogurt (4 oz nonfat, any flavor)	60	60 Cal
LUNCH		
Salad (3 oz canned tuna, 1 tsp Evoo, onions, celery)	175	
Lettuce & tomato wedges + rye bread (1 slice)	60	
Fresh fruit in season – (apple, pear, etc)	70	
Diet soda or water	0	335 Cal
SNACK		
Kashi TLC Chewy Granola Bar	140	
Coffee or tea	10	150 Cal
DINNER		
Low-Cal Beef Stew (Recipe 29 - page 146)	365	
Large tossed salad with 1½ Tbsp low-cal dressing	85	
Small whole-grain roll	80	
Water with lemon wedge	15	545 Cal
SNACK		
Graham crackers (4 squares)	120	
Coffee or tea	10	130 Cal
		1500 Cal

Cooking Daily Menu 30

BREAKFAST	Calories	Totals
Fresh sliced orange	75	
Cheerios (1 cup) + ½ cup skim milk + about 15 raisins	190	
Whole-grain toast (1 slice)	70	
Coffee	10	345 Cal
SNACK		
Fresh fruit in season (peach, plum, etc)	70	
Coffee or tea	10	80 Cal
LUNCH		
Cottage cheese (1 cup low fat)	180	
Large tossed salad with 1½ Tbsp low-cal dressing	85	
Small whole-grain roll	80	
Hot or iced tea	10	355 Cal
SNACK		
Handful unsalted mixed nuts	100	
Coffee or tea	10	110 Cal
DINNER		
Chicken with veggies (Recipe 30 - page 147)	365	
Yogurt (4 oz nonfat, any flavor)	60	
Water with lemon wedge	15	440 Cal
SNACK		
Dark chocolate (1 oz)	150	
Coffee or tea	10	160 Cal
		1490 Cal

Cooking Daily Menu 31

BREAKFAST	Calories	Totals
Orange juice (½ cup)	50	
Shredded Wheat (1 cup) + ½ cup skim milk + ½ banana	260	
Coffee	10	320 Cal
SNACK		
Handful unsalted mixed nuts	100	
Coffee or tea	10	110 Cal
LUNCH		
Turkey frank (2 oz) with mustard & relish	150	
Hot dog bun	130	
Hot or iced tea	10	290 Cal
SNACK		
Yogurt (4 oz nonfat, any flavor)	60	
Coffee or tea	10	70 Cal
DINNER		
Pasta e Fagioli (Recipe 31 - page 148)	300	
Large tossed salad with 1½ Tbsp low-cal dressing	85	
Italian or French bread (1 slice)	80	
Glass of red wine (4 oz)	100	
Water with lemon wedge	15	580 Cal
SNACK		
Graham crackers (4 squares)	120	
Coffee or tea	10	130 Cal
		1500 Cal

Cooking Daily Menu 32

BREAKFAST	Calories	Totals
Fresh or frozen strawberries (½ cup)	25	
French toasted English Muffin (Recipe 3 - page 119)	270	
Light syrup (1 Tbsp)	30	
Coffee	10	335 Cal
SNACK		
Yogurt (4 oz nonfat, any flavor)	60	
Coffee or tea	10	70 Cal
LUNCH		
Chicken, broccoli & cheddar*	270	
Hot or iced tea	10	280 Cal
* Hot Pockets wrap		
SNACK		
Handful unsalted mixed nuts	100	
Coffee or tea	10	110 Cal
DINNER		
Beef Kebob with veggies (Recipe 32 - page 149)	390	
Baked potato (medium)	100	
Fresh fruit in season (apple, pear, etc)	70	
Water with lemon wedge	15	575 Cal
SNACK		
Graham crackers (4 squares)	120	
Coffee or tea	10	130 Cal
		1500 Cal

Cooking Daily Menu 33

BREAKFAST	Calories	Totals
Orange juice (½ cup)	50	
Kashi GoLean (1 cup) + ½ cup skim milk + ½ banana	235	
Coffee	10	295 Cal
SNACK		
Fresh fruit in season (apple, peach, etc)	70	
Coffee or tea	10	80 Cal
LUNCH		
Soup (Appendix B - page 172)	100	
Small whole-grain roll	80	
Lettuce and sliced tomato with 1 Tbsp low-cal	45	
Unsweetened cinnamon-apple sauce (½ cup)	45	
Hot or iced tea	10	280 Cal
SNACK		
Popcorn Mini Bag	110	
Coffee or tea	10	120 Cal
DINNER		
Baked Haddock (Recipe 33 - page 150)	420	
Large tossed salad with 1½ Tbsp low-cal dressing	85	
Glass of red wine (4 oz)	100	
Hot or iced tea	10	615 Cal
SNACK		
100-Calorie Pack Cookies	100	
Coffee or tea	10	110 Cal
		1500 Cal

Cooking Daily Menu 34

BREAKFAST	Calories	Totals
Cantaloupe (½ medium)	50	
Perfect egg (Recipe 8a - page 124)	80	
Turkey bacon (2 slices)	70	
Toasted raisin bread (1 slice)	75	
Coffee	10	285 Cal
SNACK		
Yogurt (4 oz nonfat, any flavor)	60	
Coffee or tea	10	70 Cal
LUNCH		
Soup (Appendix B - page 172)	180	
Lettuce & tomato sandwich (1 Tbsp light mayo)	180	
Water with lemon wedge	15	375 Cal
SNACK		
Handful unsalted mixed nuts	100	
Coffee or tea	10	110 Cal
DINNER		
Chicken Cacciatore (Recipe 34a - page 151)	310	
Italian or French bread (1 slice)	80	
Glass of red wine (4 oz)	100	
Water with lemon wedge	15	505 Cal
SNACK		
Blueberry muffin (Recipe 34b - page 152)	145	
Coffee or tea	10	155 Cal
		1500 Cal

Cooking Daily Menu 35

BREAKFAST	Calories	Totals
Grapefruit (½)	75	
Cheerios (1 cup) + ½ cup skim milk + about 15 raisins	190	
Coffee	10	275 Cal
SNACK		
Fresh fruit in season (apple, plum, etc)	70	70 Cal
LUNCH		
Cottage cheese (1 cup low fat)	180	
Large tossed salad with 1½ Tbsp low-cal dressing	85	
Small whole-grain roll	80	
Hot or iced tea	10	355 Cal
SNACK		
Handful unsalted mixed nuts	100	
Coffee or tea	10	110 Cal
DINNER		
Poached Cod (Recipe 35 - page 153)	275	
Grilled potatoes	100	
Grilled cherry tomatoes	45	
Spinach (½ cup) steamed with garlic & drizzled	50	
Whole-grain bread (1 slice)	70	
Water	0	540 Cal
SNACK		
Blueberry muffin	145	
Coffee or tea	10	155 Cal
		1505 Cal

Cooking Daily Menu 36

BREAKFAST	Calories	Totals
Fresh orange sliced	75	
Soft-boiled egg	80	
Whole grain toast (2 slices)	140	
Coffee	10	305 Cal
SNACK		
Yogurt (4 oz nonfat, any flavor)	60	
Coffee or tea	10	70 Cal
LUNCH		
Salad – 3 oz canned salmon, 1 tsp Evoo, onions & celery	200	
Lettuce & tomato wedges	20	
Rye bread (1 slice)	70	
Fresh fruit in season (apple, peach, etc)	70	
Coffee or tea	10	370 Cal
SNACK		
Handful unsalted mixed nuts	100	
Coffee or tea	10	110 Cal
DINNER		
Chicken Piccata (Recipe 36 - page 154)	270	
Brown rice (½ cup – after cooking)	100	
Large tossed salad with 1½ Tbsp low-cal dressing	85	
Water	0	455 Cal
SNACK		
Graham crackers (4 squares)	120	
Skim milk (6 oz)	70	190 Cal
		1500 Cal

Cooking Daily Menu 37

BREAKFAST	Calories	Totals
Cantaloupe (½ medium)	50	
Wheaties (¾ cup) + ½ cup skim milk + ½ banana	190	
Whole grain toast (1 slice)	70	
Coffee	10	320 Cal
SNACK		
Handful unsalted mixed nuts	100	
Coffee or tea	10	110 Cal
LUNCH		
Ham (2 oz) with mustard on 2 slices rye bread	290	
Pickle spear	0	
Small bunch of grapes	65	
Hot or iced tea	10	365 Cal
SNACK		
Yogurt (4 oz nonfat, any flavor)	60	
Coffee or tea	10	70 Cal
DINNER		
Beans and Greens Salad (Recipe 37 - page 155)	260	
Whole-grain bread (1 slice)	70	
Baked potato (medium)	100	
Water with lemon wedge	15	515 Cal
SNACK		
100-Calorie Pack Cookies	100	
Coffee or tea	10	110 Cal
		1490 Cal

Cooking Daily Menu 38

BREAKFAST	Calories	Totals
Fresh or frozen strawberries (1 cup)	25	
French toasted English Muffin (Recipe 3 - page 119)	270	
Light syrup (1 Tbsp)	30	
Coffee	10	335 Cal
SNACK		
Fresh fruit in season (pear, plum, etc)	70	
Coffee or tea	10	80 Cal
LUNCH		
Soup (Appendix B - page 172)	90	
BLT sandwich (2 slices turkey bacon, 1 Tbsp light	245	
Pickle spear	0	
Water	0	335 Cal
SNACK		
Handful unsalted mixed nuts	100	100 Cal
DINNER		
Pan-fried Sole (Recipe 38 - page 156)	325	
Large tossed salad with 1½ Tbsp low-cal dressing	85	
Whole-grain bread (1 slice)	70	
Water	0	480 Cal
SNACK		
Skinny Cow Ice Cream Sandwich	160	
Coffee or tea	10	170 Cal
		1500 Cal

BREAKFAST	Calories	Totals
Grapefruit (½)	75	
Cheerios (1 cup) + ½ cup skim milk + about 15 raisins	190	
Coffee	10	**275 Cal**
## SNACK		
Fresh fruit in season (peach, plum, etc)	70	
Coffee or tea	10	**80 Cal**
## LUNCH		
Cottage cheese (1 cup low fat)	180	
Large tossed salad with 1½ Tbsp low-cal dressing	85	
Small whole-grain roll	80	
Hot or iced tea	10	**355 Cal**
## SNACK		
Handful unsalted mixed nuts	100	
Coffee or tea	10	**110 Cal**
## DINNER		
Beef steak strips (Recipe 39 - page 157)	330	
Steamed spinach (½ cup)	25	
Baked potato (medium)	100	
Whole-grain bread (1 slice)	70	
Water	0	**525 Cal**
## SNACK		
Blueberry muffin	145	
Coffee or tea	10	**155 Cal**
		1500 Cal

<h2 align="center"><u>Cooking Daily Menu 40</u></h2>

BREAKFAST	Calories	Totals
Cantaloupe (½ medium)	50	
Fried eggs (2 eggs)	160	
Toasted whole-grain bread (2 slices)	140	
Coffee	10	360 Cal
SNACK		
Yogurt (4 oz nonfat, any flavor)	60	
Coffee or tea	10	70 Cal
LUNCH		
Soup (Appendix B - page 172)	190	
Hard whole-grain roll (medium)	80	
Lettuce & tomato slices	20	
Water with lemon wedge	15	305 Cal
SNACK		
Fresh fruit in season (apple, peach, etc)	70	
Coffee or tea	10	80 Cal
DINNER		
Grilled scallops (Recipe 40 - page 158)	210	
Grilled polenta (Recipe 40)	125	
Mushroom-steamed green beans-red onion (Recipe 40)	45	
Grilled asparagus (Recipe 40)	10	
Large tossed salad with 1½ Tbsp low-cal dressing	85	
Glass of wine (4 oz)	100	
Water	0	575 Cal
SNACK		
100-Calorie Pack Cookies	100	
Coffee or tea	10	110 Cal
		1500 Cal

Cooking Daily Menu 41

BREAKFAST	Calories	Totals
Tomato juice (½ cup)	20	
Kashi GoLean (1 cup) + ½ cup skim milk + ½ banana	235	
Coffee	10	265 Cal
SNACK		
Fresh fruit in season (apple, plum, etc)	70	70 Cal
LUNCH		
Soup (Appendix B - page 172)	100	
Small whole-grain roll	80	
Lettuce & sliced tomato w 1 Tbsp low-cal dressing	45	
Unsweetened cinnamon-apple sauce (½ cup)	45	
Hot or iced tea	10	280 Cal
SNACK		
Popcorn Mini Bag	110	
Coffee or tea	10	120 Cal
DINNER		
Grilled pork chop w orange (Recipe 41 - page 159)	470	
Wild rice (¼ cup – after cooking)	50	
Asparagus (7 spear cooked & drained)	20	
Large tossed salad with 1½ Tbsp low-cal dressing	70	
Water	0	610 Cal
SNACK		
Blueberry muffin	145	
Coffee or tea	10	155 Cal
		1500 Cal

<u>Cooking Daily Menu 42</u>

<u>BREAKFAST</u>	**<u>Calories</u>**	**<u>Totals</u>**
Cantaloupe (½ medium)	50	
Smoothie (Recipe 42a - page 160)	220	
Coffee	10	**280 Cal**
<u>SNACK</u>		
Handful unsalted mixed nuts	100	**100 Cal**
<u>LUNCH</u>		
Turkey breast (2 oz) on 2 slices whole-grain bread	245	
Lettuce, tomato and 1 Tbsp light mayo	35	
Pickle spear	0	
Water with lemon wedge	10	**290 Cal**
<u>SNACK</u>		
100-Calorie Pack Cookies	100	
Coffee or tea	10	**110 Cal**
<u>DINNER</u>		
Pasta Salad (Recipe 42b - Page 161)	370	
Italian or French bread (1 slice)	80	
Glass of red wine (4 oz)	100	
Water with lemon wedge	15	**565 Cal**
<u>SNACK</u>		
Blueberry muffin	145	
Coffee or tea	10	**155 Cal**
		1500 Cal

Cooking Daily Menu 43

BREAKFAST	Calories	Totals
Fresh or frozen strawberries (½ cup)	25	
French toasted English Muffin (Recipe 3 - page 119)	270	
Light syrup (1½ Tbsp)	45	
Coffee	10	350 Cal
SNACK		
Yogurt (4 oz – nonfat, any flavor)	60	
Coffee or tea	10	70 Cal
LUNCH		
Salad (3 oz canned tuna, 1 tsp Evoo, onions, celery)	175	
Lettuce & tomato wedges	20	
Rye bread (1 slice)	70	
Fresh fruit in season (apple, peach, etc)	70	
Coffee or tea	10	345 Cal
SNACK		
Fresh fruit in season (apple, pear, etc)	70	
Coffee or tea	10	80 Cal
DINNER		
Beef Burgundy (Recipe 43 - page 162)	350	
Large tossed salad with 1½ Tbsp low-cal dressing	85	
Whole-grain bread (1 slice)	70	
Water with lemon wedge	15	520 Cal
SNACK		
Graham crackers (4 squares)	120	
Coffee or tea	10	130 Cal
		1495 Cal

<u>Cooking Daily Menu 44</u>

BREAKFAST	Calories	Totals
Grapefruit (½)	75	
Perfect egg (See Recipe 8a - page 105)	80	
Turkey bacon (1 slice)	35	
Whole grain toast (1 slice)	70	
Coffee	10	270 Cal
SNACK		
Yogurt (4 oz nonfat, any flavor)	60	
Coffee or tea	10	70 Cal
LUNCH		
Ham (2 oz) with mustard on 2 slices rye bread	290	
Pickle spear	0	
Gelatin dessert (unsweetened)	10	
Hot or iced tea	10	310 Cal
SNACK		
Fresh fruit in season (peach, plum, etc)	70	
Coffee or tea	10	80 Cal
DINNER		
Chicken cutlet (Recipe 44 - page 163)	450	
One medium baked potato	100	
Large tossed salad with 1½ Tbsp low-cal dressing*	85	
Water with lemon wedge	15	650 Cal
* Note Much of salad is on plate with cutlet.		
SNACK		
Skinny Cow Fudge Ice Cream Bar	110	
Coffee or tea	10	120 Cal
		1500 Cal

Cooking Daily Menu 45

BREAKFAST	Calories	Totals
Grapefruit (½)	75	
Cheerios (1 cup) + ½ cup skim milk	190	
Coffee	10	275 Cal
SNACK		
Fresh fruit in season (apple, plum, etc)	70	70 Cal
LUNCH		
Cottage cheese (1 cup low fat)	180	
Tossed salad with 1½ Tbsp low-cal dressing	85	
Small whole-grain roll	80	
Hot or iced tea	10	355 Cal
SNACK		
Handful unsalted mixed nuts	100	
Coffee or tea	10	110 Cal
DINNER		
Personal-Size Meat Loaf (Recipe 45 - page 164)	410	
Brown rice (½ cup – after cooking)	100	
Green beans - steamed	30	
Water	0	540 Cal
SNACK		
Blueberry muffin	145	
Coffee or tea	10	155 Cal
		1505 Cal

Recipes and Diet Tips

Recipe 1

<u>Chicken with Peppers & Onions</u>

    4 boneless and skinless chicken breasts (5 oz each)

Coat the chicken breasts in a bottled barbeque sauce. Prepare medium-hot fire on well-oiled grill. Place breasts on grill, turning them every 4 minutes, for 10 to 12 minutes, or until done. (To check if breasts are done, the meat should be moist and white with no sign of pink when you cut into the breast.) Salt and pepper to taste.

    2 medium red peppers, sliced

    1 medium onion, sliced

Place peppers and onions in pan with 2 tablespoons fat-free chicken stock. Sauté until stock is reduced. Spray pan lightly with non-stick cooking oil and cook another 2 minutes. Salt and pepper to taste.

<u>Serves 4</u>. About 250 Calories per serving (for chicken only).

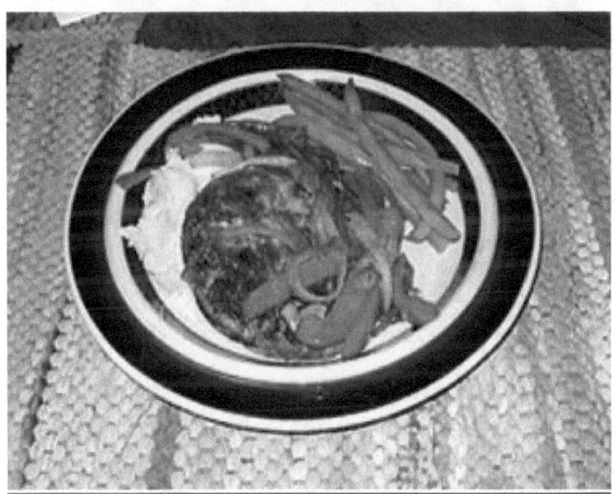

<u>Diet Tip of the Day:</u> Weight Loss – take it one meal, one workout, one day at a time. Just think of where you'll be in 60 days!

Recipe 2

<u>Baked Herb-Crusted Cod</u>

    4 cod fish fillets (4 to 5 ounces each)
    2 tablespoons flour
    2 tablespoons cornmeal
    2 tablespoons minced fresh herbs
    2 teaspoons lemon juice

Sprinkle cod with lemon juice. Mix flour, cornmeal and herbs and dust the cod with the cornmeal-herb mixture. Bake in oven at 375 °F for 10 minutes. Add salt and black pepper to taste.

<u>Serves 4</u>. One serving is about 230 Calories (for cod only).

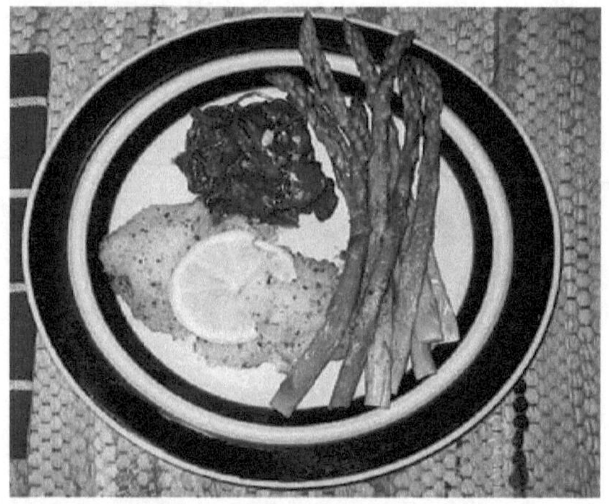

<u>Diet Tip of the Day:</u>. A **reducing diet is best supervised by a physician**. This is especially true when a great deal of weight needs to be lost, or if you have an ailment or a history of medical problems.

Recipe 3

French-Toasted English Muffin

> 6 whole grain light English muffins, sliced in half
> 4 eggs
> 2 cups skim milk
> 2 teaspoons vanilla
> A dash of cinnamon

In a medium bowl, beat together eggs and skim milk. Add vanilla and cinnamon. Slice English muffins into halves and saturate slices in egg mixture. In a non-stick skillet coated with cooking spray, cook muffins until both sides are golden brown. Dust lightly with confectionary sugar. Serve hot or keep in an oven or warmer at 200 ºF until ready to plate. **Serves 4**. Three English muffin slices per serving. Serving is 270 Calories.

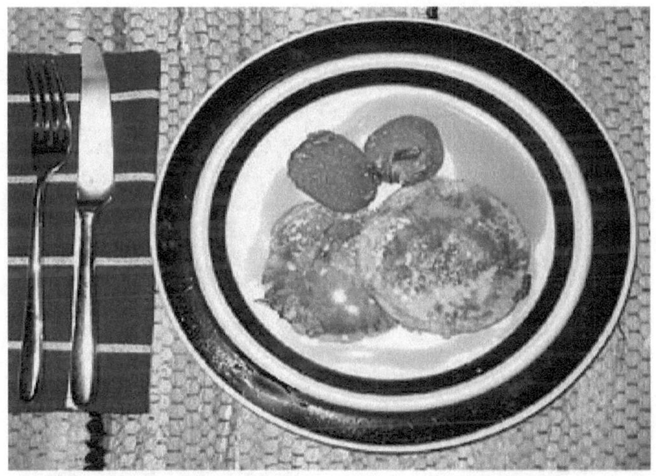

Diet Tip of the Day: "Eat Slowly" This is especially vital when you are trying to lose weight. If you are someone who eats fast, who finishes before everyone else at the table, you are not giving yourself a chance to feel full. While everyone else is still eating, you either sit there and pick, or you have seconds, taking in extra calories you could avoid if you would just slow down.

Recipe 4

<u>Carrie's Low-Cal Meat Loaf</u>

    ½ pound ground white meat turkey
    ½ pound ground beef (about 60% lean)
    1 large egg
    ½ cup skim milk
    ¼ cup bread crumbs
    ¼ cup ketchup
    ¼ cup chopped carrots
    ¼ cup chopped onion

In a medium bowl, combine all ingredients. Add salt and pepper to taste.
Mix until blended and form into a loaf. Place loaf into oven preheated to
350 °F. Bake until an instant-read thermometer inserted in the center of the
loaf reads 160 °F. This should take about one hour.

Shown below is meat loaf, acorn squash (baked with 1 teaspoon of maple
syrup). Also shown is steamed spinach drizzled with extra-virgin olive oil.
<u>Serves 5</u>. About 290 Calories per serving (for meat loaf only). Note:
reserve half a serving of the meat loaf which is to be eaten for lunch on
Day 6.

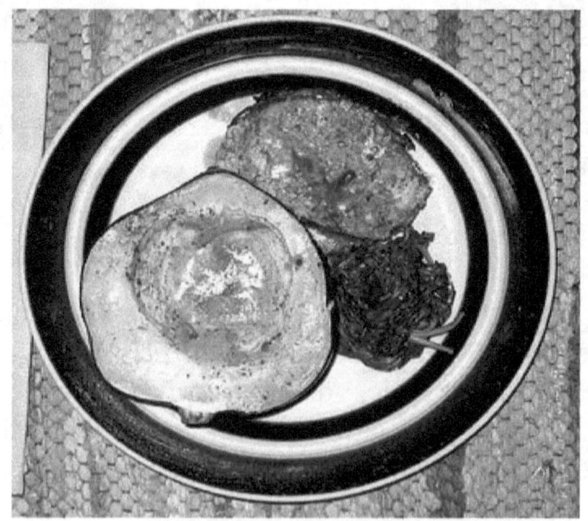

<u>Diet Tip of the Day:</u>   **Take a daily multi-vitamin/mineral supplement.**
This is very important when you're on a diet – as a kind of insurance
policy.

<u>Veal with Mushrooms & Tomato</u>

- ½ pound spaghetti
- ¾ pound veal cutlets
- 8 ounces sliced mushrooms
- 2 tablespoon olive oil, divided
- 2 tablespoons flour
- 3 green onions, small, sliced
- ½ cup chicken broth
- 14.5-ounce can of diced tomatoes

Pound veal to about ¼-inch thickness. Rinse, pat dry and cut into 2-inch pieces. Heat 1 tablespoon olive oil in large nonstick skillet over medium heat. Add mushrooms and cook, stirring, until lightly browned. Remove and set aside.

Season veal with salt and pepper and coat lightly with flour. Add remaining olive oil to skillet and cook veal over medium heat for about 2 minutes on each side, or until browned. Add the green onions and cook for 1 minute longer. Add chicken broth and cook, uncovered, for 5 minutes. Add tomatoes; cover and simmer for 3 to 5 minutes. Serve over spaghetti cooked per package directions.

<u>Serves 4</u>. 520 Calories per serving (includes spaghetti)

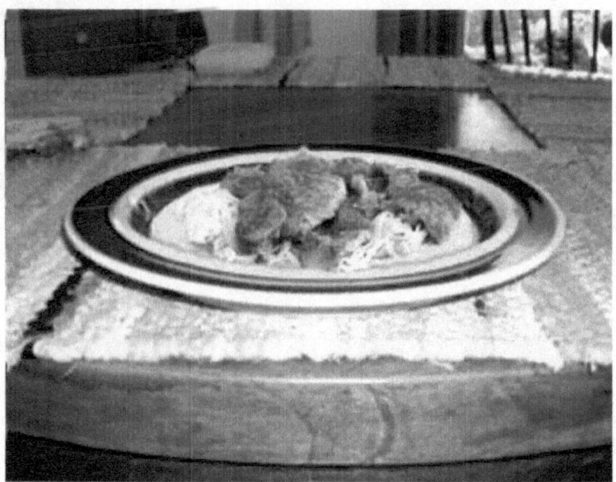

<u>Diet Tip of the Day:</u> Successful weight loss and subsequent weight maintenance **requires knowledge, desire and discipline**. Avoid the latest fad diets. Instead, take the time to develop a true understanding of weight control and then change your eating and activity habits accordingly.

Recipe 6

<u>Grandma's Pizza</u>

The following is a pizza recipe used by Gail Johnson's Italian grandmother. She was from a small mountain village located between Rome and Naples.

Pizza dough: To save time use prepared dough, preferably whole grain. To start, flour a large cutting board. Divide one pound of prepared pizza dough into four parts. Roll out each dough ball as thin as possible.

Tomato sauce: Sauté ½ small onion, chopped fine, in 1 teaspoon olive oil. Add two finely chopped garlic cloves, 1½ cups chopped plum tomatoes and ½ teaspoon chopped fresh oregano. Stir and cook about 5 minutes on a low flame.

Pizza preparation & cooking: On each pizza, spread evenly ¼ cup of the tomato sauce. Add ½ ounce of shredded part-skim mozzarella cheese, 1 teaspoon Parmesan cheese, 3 slices of a Portobello mushroom, some torn fresh basil, and drizzle with extra-virgin olive oil. Put pizzas on a pan and place in 475 ºF oven for about 15 to 20 minutes, or until crust is crisp and cheese is just melting. (Freeze left over sauce for use on Day 13.)

<u>Serves 4</u>.   Each pizza contains approximately 350 Calories.

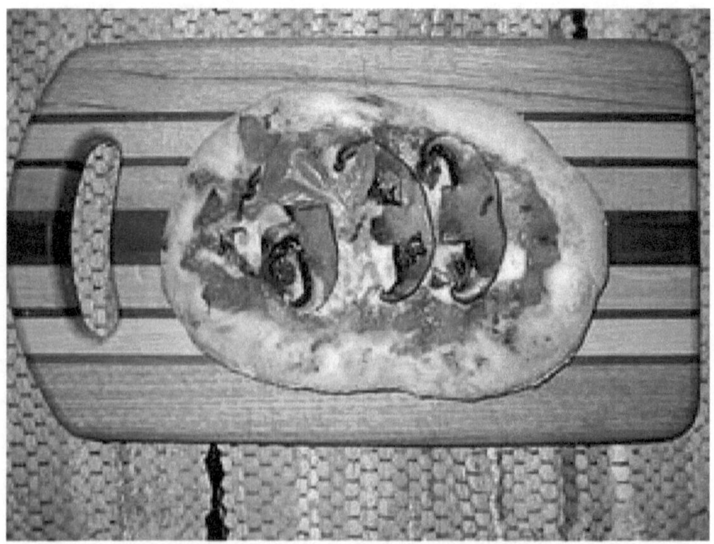

<u>Diet Tip of the Day:</u> For **life-long weight control** take a vigorous 30 to 60 minute walk everyday! That's right – everyday. Make exercise a nonflexible top priority part of your life. When it comes to exercise the key words are consistent, persistent, unyielding, dogged. Get the point?

126

Recipe 7

<u>Baked Salmon with Salsa</u>

This is a simple, straight-forward recipe. The advantage of a simple recipe is there are no hidden calories.

    4   5 oz salmon fillets

    6   tablespoons bottled tomato-pepper salsa

Brown salmon fillets in non-stick pan and then place them in a baking dish. Cook fillets in an oven preheated to 350 ºF for about 10 minutes. Plate the salmon. Stir bottled tomato-pepper salsa and spoon it over the salmon. <u>Serves 4</u>. One salmon fillet is about 215 Calories.

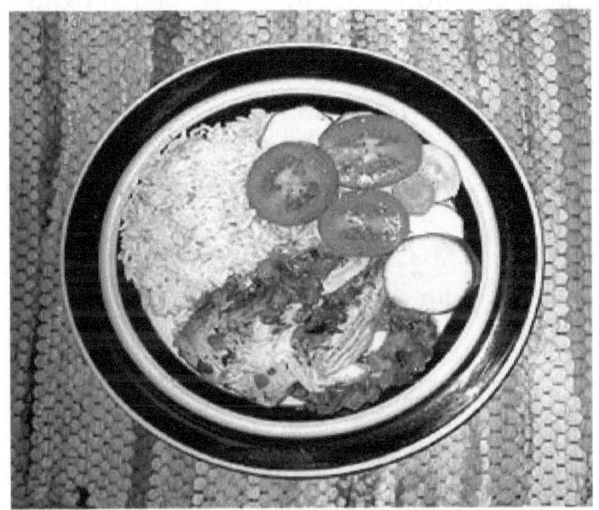

<u>Diet Tip of the Day:</u> Hunger is your body's way of telling you that you need calories. But **when you're done eating, you should feel better – satisfied but not stuffed**.

Recipe 8a

<u>The Perfect Egg</u>

Why perfect? Because it's cooked with no added fat, and a perfect egg is low calorie, nutritious and delicious. It takes about one minute to prepare - and there is virtually no clean up afterwards. It's perfect for busy people on the go, or for anyone who wants a quick, easy nutritious breakfast. For best results cook the egg in a well-glazed (shinny and smooth), microwave safe, 4-inch diameter cup with straight sides and a flat bottom.

<u>Step 1</u>: In the microwave-safe cup, beat an extra-large egg with about 2 teaspoons of added water for easy clean up.

<u>Step 2</u>: Place cup in microwave at full power for approximately 40 seconds, or until the egg begins to rise, gets fluffy and most of the added water has evaporated. (The actually cooking time will depend on how powerful your microwave is.) Salt and pepper to taste.

<u>Step 3</u>: Remove cup from the microwave and slide the egg onto a slice of whole-grain toast, (or as shown in the photo on a toasted bagel). Salt and pepper to taste.

<u>**Serves 1**</u>: Perfect Egg is 80 Calories. When a Perfect Egg is eaten with a slice of whole grain toast the calorie total is about 150.

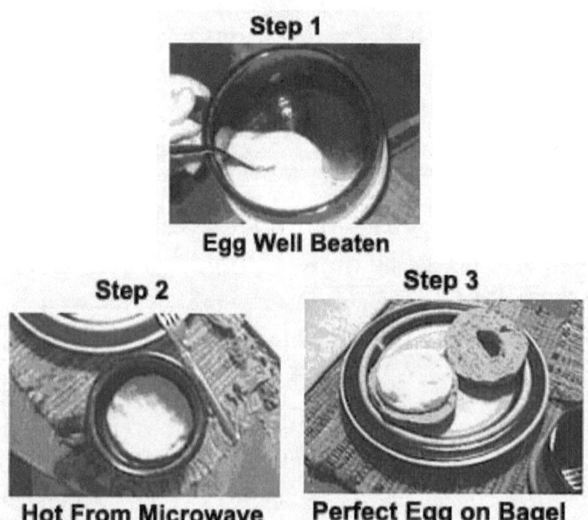

<u>**Diet Tip of the Day:**</u> The average egg has only 210 mg of cholesterol (found in the yoke), contains 80 calories, many vitamins many minerals. If you're healthy and your LDL blood cholesterol level is low, many experts feel you can safely eat one egg per day.

Veggie Burger

Vegetable-based burgers can be purchased at your local supermarket. Patties of a veggie burger are made from either vegetables, soy, nuts, mushrooms, textured vegetable protein, dairy, or a combination of these foods.

In the U.S., two popular veggie burgers are the Boca Burger and Gardenburger. The Boca Burger is made chiefly from soy protein and grain gluten. (Boca Burger patties are 2.5 oz each and range from 60 to 60 Calories.) The original Gardenburger is made from mushrooms, onions, brown rice, rolled oats, cheese, and spices. (Gardenburger patties are 2.5 oz each and about 100 Calories.)

To prepare, follow package directions. The version shown below has an added slice of low-fat cheddar cheese. The lettuce, tomato and ketchup shown actually add very few extra calories.

The veggie burger patty plus low-fat cheese amounts to approximately 150 Calories. Add a seeded roll and the total rises to 290 Calories.

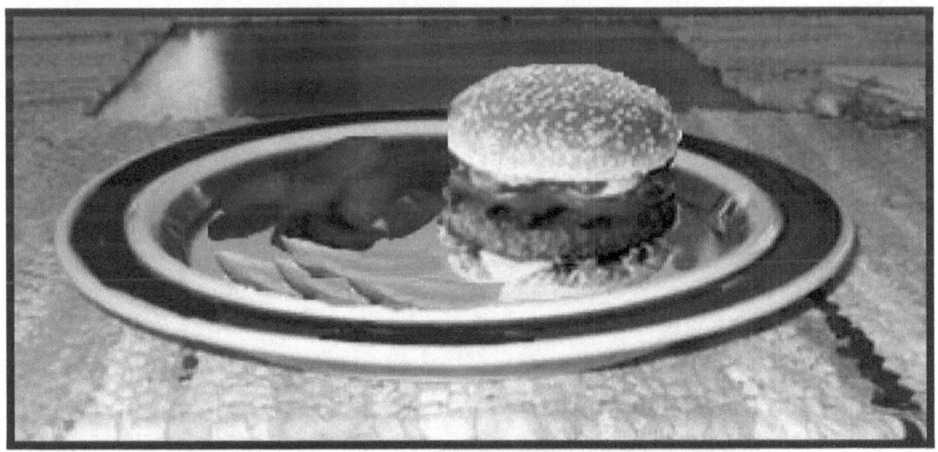

Diet Tip of the Day: **Drink lots of water** – about 8 glasses per day when you're trying to lose weight. Add a slice of lemon to make it more interesting. Often, when you think you're hungry, you are just thirsty. So, next time you crave a snack, drink some water first and see if that does it for you.

Recipe 9

<u>Wild Blueberry Pancakes</u>

This recipe makes a relatively low calorie, wholesome batch of delicious wild blueberry-whole grain-buttermilk pancakes.

    1 cup whole-grain flour
    1 cup buttermilk
    1 egg
    1 tablespoon vegetable oil
    1 teaspoon baking powder
    ½ teaspoon baking soda

Stir ingredients until blended. Add ¾ cup fresh of frozen blueberries and gently stir. Using medium heat, preheat a non-stick skillet coated with cooking spray. Pour slightly less than ¼ cup of batter onto skillet per pancake. Cook slowly until bubbles break on surface of pancake. Turn and cook until other side is lightly browned.

Makes 8 pancakes. Pictured below are wild-blueberry pancakes with two slices of turkey bacon.

<u>**Serves 4**</u>. Each pancake is about 95 Calories

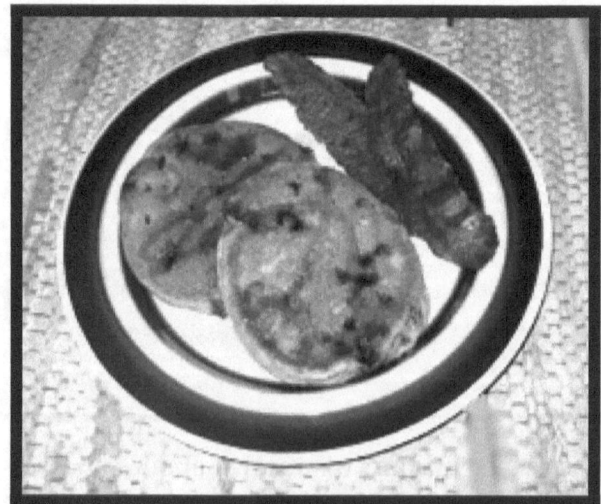

Turkey bacon allowable only on 1500 and 1800 Calorie diets.

<u>**Diet Tip of the Day:**</u> Most experts associate eating breakfast with successful weight loss.

Recipe 10

Artichoke-Bean Salad

        19-ounce can white kidney beans
        10 artichoke hearts, quartered
        ⅓ cup chopped oregano
        ⅓ cup chopped parsley
        3 cloves garlic, chopped
        1 lemon, juiced

Combine ingredients in medium-size bowl. Stir in ¼ cup extra-virgin olive oil. Salt and black pepper to taste.

Serves 6. Approximately 190 Calories per serving.

Pictured on the plate below is the artichoke-bean salad as a side dish with two grilled chicken sausage links, tomato salsa and steamed green beans. Incidentally, this artichoke-bean combination over mixed salad greens served with a whole-grain bread makes a delicious, nutritious and reasonable low-calorie main course.

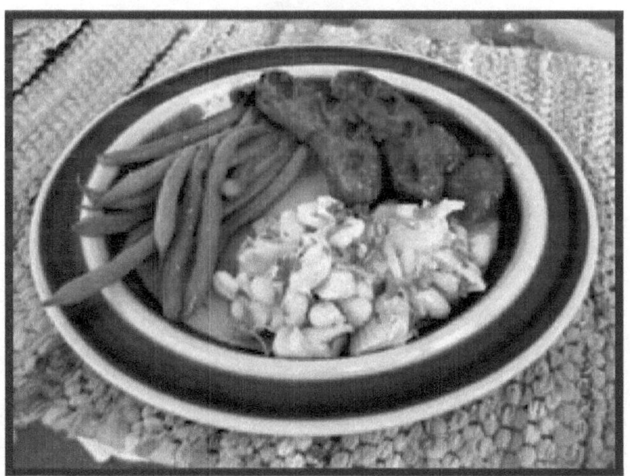

Diet Tip of the Day: Before you go to a **party**, have a small meal, such as a hardboiled egg, an apple, and a thirst quencher (like water, tea, seltzer, or diet soda). This will take the edge off your appetite and make it easier to resist the high-calorie goodies.

Recipe 11

<u>Pasta with Marinara Sauce</u>

Prepare the sauce as you did for the Day 6 pizza (see page 113). But because the pizza sauce is a bit too thick, we add ¼ cup of pasta liquid to thin it. (The spiral pasta profile shown below is called fusilli, a very popular pasta shape because all those ridges hold buckets of tomato sauce.)

    ½ pound <u>whole-grain</u> pasta
    ¼ teaspoon salt

Prepare the marinara tomato sauce as per Day 6 sauce but dilute it with ¼ cup of today's pasta liquid.

Bring 2 quarts of lightly salted water to a boil. Add pasta and stir occasionally (to keep pasta from sticking to the bottom of the pot). Keep water boiling and cook until pasta are "al dente." (Cooking time is approximately 9 minutes.) Drain pasta, add marinara sauce and serve hot. **Serves 4.** One serving is about 225 Calories.

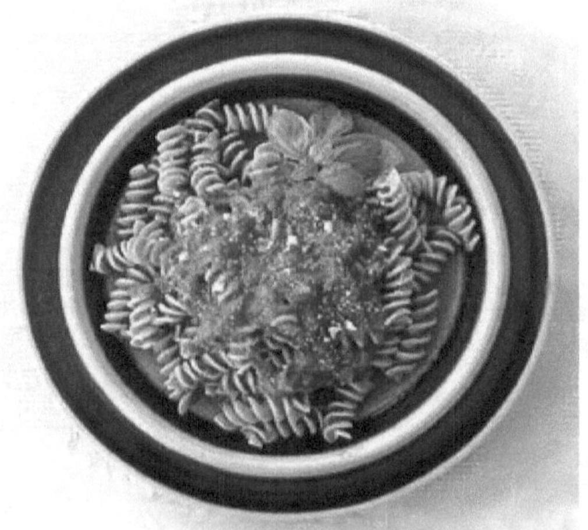

<u>**Diet Tip of the Day:**</u> **Beware of alcoholic beverages**. Beer has about 13 Calories per ounce, wine 25 Calories per ounce and whiskey a whopping 71 Calories per ounce.

London Broil

   1 lb boneless flank steak about ¾" thick, fat trimmed
   1 clove garlic
   1 teaspoon dry oregano

Rub each side of the flank steak with garlic. Season with oregano, salt and pepper to taste. Prepare a large non-stick skillet over high heat. Steak should sizzle when placed on hot skillet. Sear steak on one side for about 5 minutes; then turn and sear other side for about 4 minutes, or until done to preference. Check the center by making small incision. Carve into ¼-inch slices.

Serves 4. About 320 Calories per serving (for meat only).

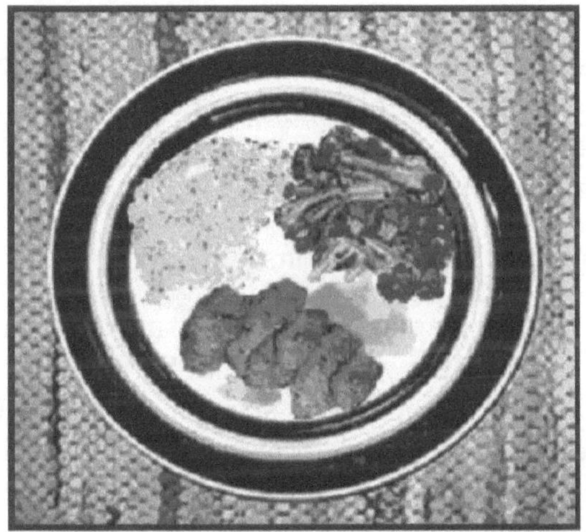

Diet Tip of the Day: Stay Busy. Most people will do anything to avoid work, housework, yard work, exercise, etc. But any kind of work burns a lot more calories than just sitting! Whatever it is you are avoiding – just go do it!

Recipe 13

<u>Red Snapper with Special Sauce</u>

  4 4-ounce red snapper fillets (salmon fillets okay)
  ½ cup white wine
  ½ cup non-fat yogurt mixed with ¼ cup mustard
  ½ pound green beans
  ¾ pint cherry tomatoes (about 20), halved
  4 teaspoons olive oil
  ¾ cup wild rice, brown rice and grain berry mix.

Brown fillets in non-stick pan. Place fillets skin side down in baking dish coated with non-stick spray. Add white wine and cook in oven preheated to 350 °F for about 15 minutes . Spoon pan juices over fillets. Salt and pepper to taste.

Place green beans in skillet. Add ¼-inch of water and cook over medium heat until water boils off. Add cherry tomatoes and olive oil. Stir well and sauté for a few minutes. (If desired, season with fresh rosemary and oregano.) Salt and pepper to taste.

Prepare rice mix per package directions

Plate red snapper fillet and spoon over yogurt-mustard sauce. Add green beans and tomato mix and the wild rice mix. Serve hot.

<u>Serves 4</u>. One plate consisting of one snapper fillet (215 Calories) with green beans and tomato mix (75 Calories) and wild rice (160 Calories) totals 450 Calories.

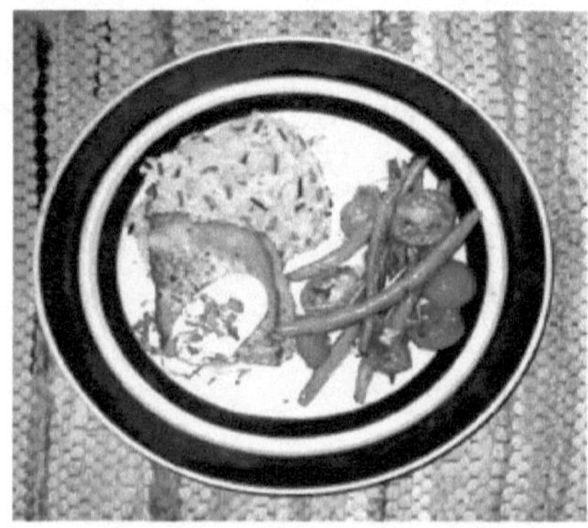

<u>Diet Tip of the Day:</u> **Don't have sweets in your house**. This makes them easier to resist. Out of sight, out of mind!

Recipe 14

<u>Cajun Chicken Salad</u>

This is a perfect after-work, quick, nutritious and delicious dinner.

- 4 boneless and skinless chicken breasts - about 5 oz each
- 4 teaspoons of bottled Cajun herb-spice mix
- 8 ounces mixed salad greens
- ¾ pint cherry tomatoes (about 20), halved
- 12 pitted black olives
- 2 tablespoons bottled light salad dressing

Brush chicken breasts lightly with olive oil. Roll breasts in Cajun herb-spice mix.

Brown breasts on non-stick oven-proof skillet. After breasts are brown, put skillet in 350 ºF oven for approximately 15 minutes, or until done. (When the breasts are done, the meat should be moist and white with no sign of pink.) Cut breasts into ½-inch slices.

Serve hot or keep in an oven or warmer at 200 ºF until ready to plate. Place chicken slices over a bed of mixed salad greens. Add tomatoes, olives and two tablespoons of your favorite low-calorie salad dressing. <u>Serves 4</u>. 330 Calories per serving

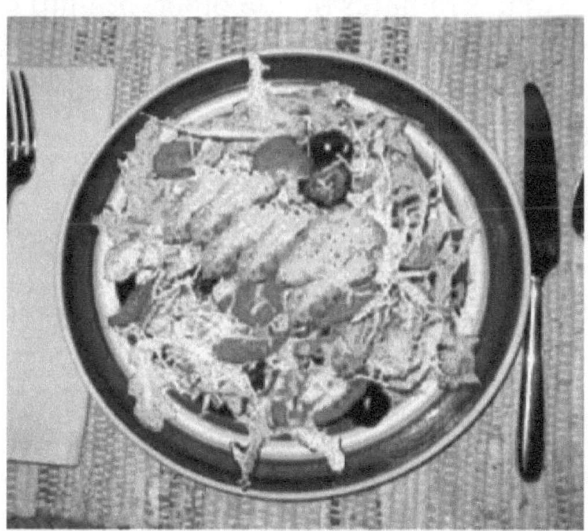

<u>Diet Tip of the Day:</u> Hot or cold cereal topped with fruit, and fat-free milk makes a nutritious, relatively low-calorie meal anytime.

<h1 style="text-align:center">Recipe 15</h1>

<u>Grilled Swordfish</u>

    1¼ pounds swordfish
    1 bottle citrus-herb marinade
    ¾ pint cherry tomatoes (about 20), halved
    4 medium potatoes
    2 cups fresh spinach
    1 teaspoon rosemary & juice of ¼ lemon
    2 teaspoon extra-virgin olive oil, divided

Steam spinach with garlic and drizzle with about 1 teaspoon extra-virgin olive oil.

Cut potatoes in medium-size pieces and sprinkle with lemon juice, add rosemary, salt and black pepper. Place potatoes on grill for about 10 minutes, turning occasionally.

Toss cherry tomatoes in remaining extra-virgin olive oil. Add fresh oregano, salt and black pepper. Place on heavy-duty aluminum foil, seal and grill for about 3 minutes.

Marinade swordfish in citrus-herb vinaigrette. Grill on hot fire for about 5 minutes on one side and 3 minutes on the other, or until done as desired. <u>**Serves 4**</u>. One plate of grilled swordfish (250 Calories) with potatoes (100 Calories), cherry tomatoes (45 Calories) and steamed spinach (50 Calories) totals 445 Calories.

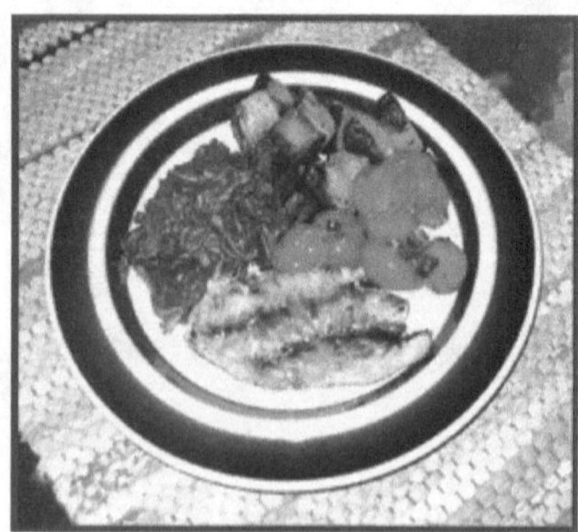

<u>**Diet Tip of the Day:**</u> **Slow weight loss is healthier,** is more likely to be permanent and is easier to sustain over the long haul. When it comes to weight loss, don't be in a hurry!

Recipe 16

<u>Quick Pasta alla Puttanesca</u>

This famous pasta dish originated in Naples Italy. Puttanesca means "ladies of the night." Although the exact origin of the name is unclear, one thing is clear: It's delicious! Here is one of many recipe versions.

> ½ pound spaghetti (whole grain preferred)
> 20 black or green pitted olives
> 14.5-oz can diced tomatoes
> 4 oz tomato sauce
> 2 tablespoon extra-virgin olive oil
> 3 cloves of garlic, chopped
> 1 tablespoon dried minced onion
> ½ teaspoon crushed red pepper flakes
> 1 tablespoon capers drained and rinsed
> ¼ cup currants

Cook spaghetti according to package directions. Drain and return spaghetti to pot; add a teaspoon extra-virgin olive oil and toss to coat.

Heat remaining olive oil in large skillet over medium-high heat. Add red pepper flakes; cook and stir 1 to 2 minutes or until sizzling. Add onion and garlic; cook and stir 1 minute. Add canned tomatoes with juice, tomato sauce, olives, currants and capers. Cook over medium-high heat, stirring frequently, until sauce is heated through.

<u>Serves 4.</u> About 345 Calories per serving

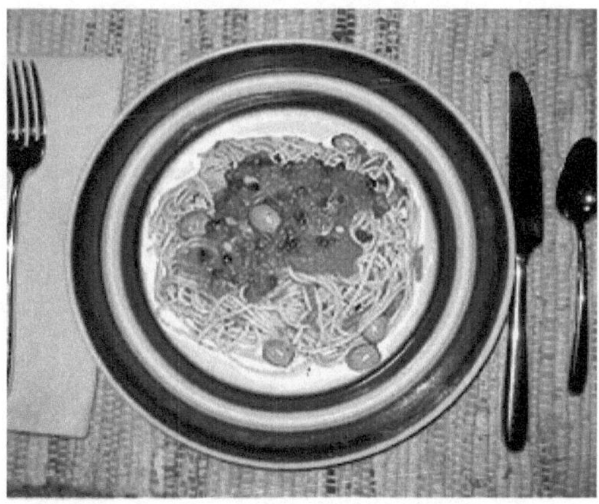

<u>Diet Tip of the Day:</u> Dilute fruit juices, such as apple juice, orange, etc. with water. This cuts the flavor slightly but really reduces calorie content.

137

Recipe 17

<u>Shrimp & Spinach Salad</u>

    2 pounds shrimp in shell
    ½ pound small green beans, trimmed
    ½ pound baby spinach leaves
    2 tablespoon lemon juice
    ¼ cup extra-virgin olive oil
    2 teaspoon minced fresh dill
    1 tablespoon minced green onion

To make vinaigrette, combine lemon juice, olive oil, dill, salt and black pepper to taste and whisk until blended. Stir in minced onion and set aside. Steam green beans and set aside.

Peel, de-vein and butterfly shrimp. Place shrimp in a bowl and add water to cover. Add 1 teaspoon of salt, and let stand for 10 minutes. Drain, rinse, drain again, and dry. Arrange shrimp in broiling pan without a rack. Brush shrimp with a little of the vinaigrette and place under preheated broiler, about 3 inches from heat. Broil about 3 to 4 minutes, turning shrimp once, or until both sides turn pink.

Remove shrimp from broiler and add remaining vinaigrette and green beans to the broiling pan. Stir to coat shrimp and beans with vinaigrette. Pour warm vinaigrette over spinach and toss quickly. Plate the spinach and arrange shrimp and green beans on top.

<u>Serves 4</u>. 310 Calories per serving.

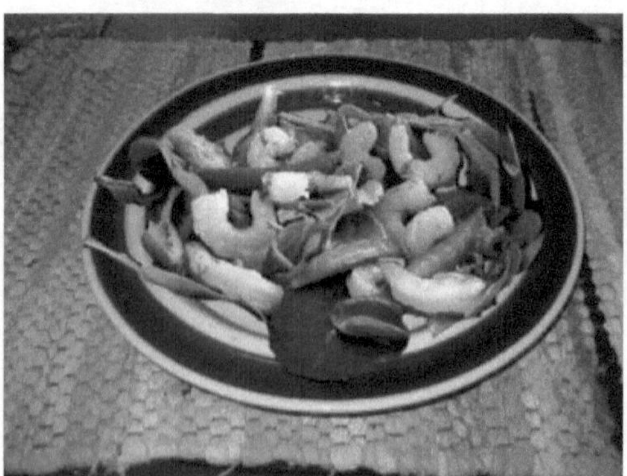

<u>Diet Tip of the Day:</u> After company leaves, have them take some of the leftover food (particularly the dessert) with them – or take the leftovers to work the next day.

Recipe 18

Pan-Broiled Hanger Steak

    1¼ pounds hanger steak, well trimmed of fat
    ¼ cup lime juice
    8 small new potatoes, peeled and halved
    ½ pint cherry tomatoes (about 15), halved

Season both sides of steak with salt and pepper and place in sealable plastic bag with lime juice. Refrigerate for about one hour.

Boil potatoes about 10 minutes. Rinse in cold water. Sauté potatoes in small amount of vegetable oil over medium-high heat until brown.

Sauté cherry tomatoes in small amount of olive oil over medium-high heat until skin begins to crack. Season with chopped fresh basil.

Heat a skillet over medium-high heat. Sear hanger steak on one side for about 5 minutes. Turn over and sear other side approximately 5 minutes (for medium done). Pour off any fat that may have accumulated. Cut into ½-inch slices.

Serves 4. About 320 Calories per serving (for the hanger steak only)

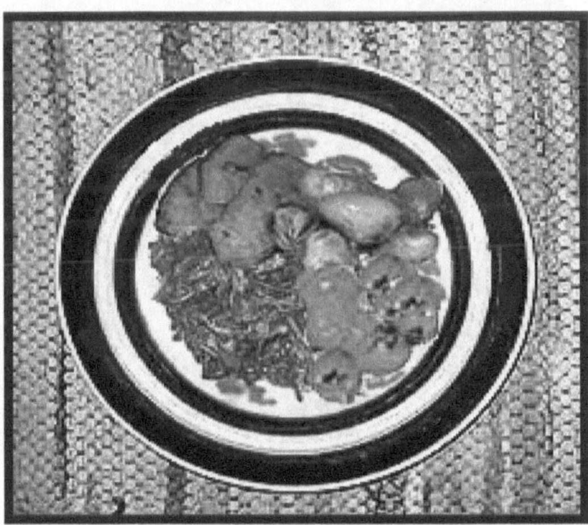

Diet Tip of the Day: If you go to a **party**, don't stand near the food! Be aware of the temptation. Make the effort, and you'll find you eat less.

Recipe 19 (This is a side dish)

<u>Four-Bean Plus Salad</u>

Note that the total caloric value of the salad will change very little, if the proportions of the bean varieties and corn are varied – according to taste.

    ½ cup canned red kidney beans, drained and rinsed
    ½ cup canned black beans, drained and rinsed
    ½ cup canned chick peas, drained and rinsed
    ½ cup canned cannelloni beans, drained and rinsed
    ½ cup canned corn, drained
    1 small red pepper, chopped
    1 small green pepper, chopped
    2 tablespoons extra-virgin olive oil
    2 tablespoons lemon juice

In a large bowl mix red kidney beans, black beans, chick peas, cannelloni beans, corn and chopped red and green peppers. Stir in olive oil and lemon juice and plate.

<u>**Serves about 6**</u>. One serving is ½ cup – with about 135 Calories per serving

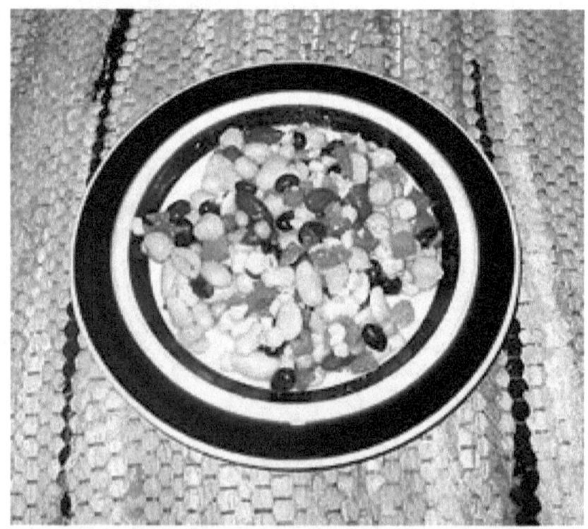

<u>**Diet Tip of the Day:**</u> Vigorous exercise doesn't necessarily stimulate you to overeat. In some cases it's just the opposite and exercise actually helps curb your appetite – immediately following a workout.

Recipe 20

<u>Beans & Greens Salad</u>

$\frac{1}{3}$ cup chopped oregano

$\frac{1}{3}$ cup chopped parsley

3 cloves garlic, chopped

1 lemon, juiced

Prepare dressing by combining above ingredients and stirring in $\frac{1}{4}$ cup extra-virgin olive oil. Salt and black pepper to taste.

$\frac{1}{2}$ pound mesclun mix

$\frac{1}{4}$ pound green beans

19-oz can garbanzo beans (chickpeas)

Arrange mesclun mix, garbanzo beans and green beans on large platter. Drizzle dressing over beans and greens.

<u>Serves 4</u>. Approximately 260 Calories per serving.

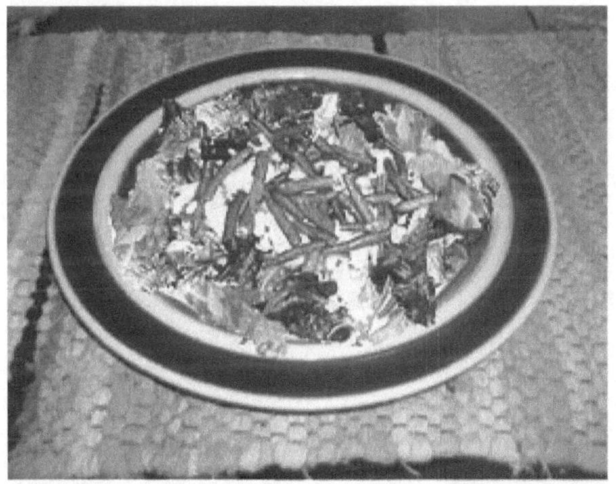

<u>Diet Tip of the Day:</u> Beans are a wonderful food but **beans are an incomplete protein**. If however beans are eaten with a whole-grain bread, the combination forms a complete protein – just as complete and nutritious as meat, poultry, or fish.

Recipe 21

<u>Grilled Scallops &Polenta</u>

    1 pound sea scallops
    ¾ cup polenta cornmeal
    ¾ cup skim milk
    1 medium portobello mushroom
    ½ pound green beans
    ¼ cup chopped red onion
    16 asparagus spear
    1 teaspoon extra-virgin olive oil

Bring 1½ cups of water and skim milk to rapid boil. Add salt to taste and slowly add polenta while stirring. Reduce heat. Continue stirring until desired consistency is reached. Pour polenta into lightly greased pan. After polenta has cooled cover and refrigerate. Cut chilled polenta into 4 pieces. Grill on medium-hot fire – about two minutes on each side.

Brush portobello mushroom and asparagus spear with olive oil and place on grill for about 3 minutes on each side.

Grill scallops on medium-hot fire. Turn after two minutes or when first side turns opaque. Grill until second side turns opaque – about another 2 minutes. Don't overcook but test a scallop by cutting to make sure it's cooked through. Salt and pepper to taste.

<u>Serves 4.</u> The food on the plate pictured below totals about 380 Calories.

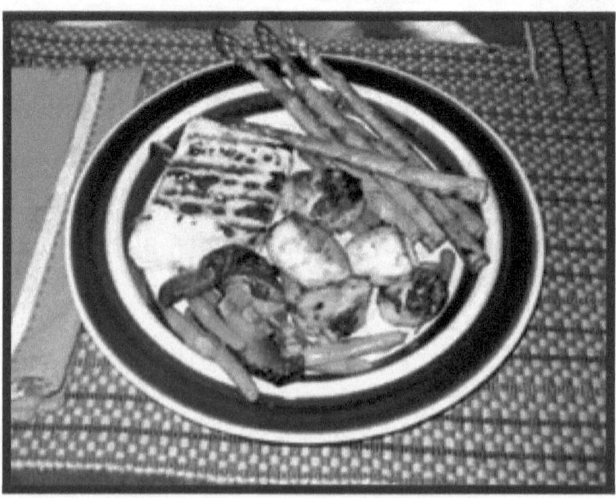

<u>Diet Tip of the Day:</u> To have better control of what you eat **bring your lunch to work**.

Recipe 22

<u>Fettuccine in Summer Sauce</u>

This sauce is often served in the summer because it's lighter than what is usually dished up with pasta. But despite its name the sauce is wonderful year round.

> ½ lb fettuccine
> 8 oz fresh asparagus, trimmed & cut in 2-inch pieces
> ¾ pint cherry tomatoes (about 20), halved
> 2 Tbsp plus 1 tsp extra-virgin olive oil, divided
> 2 cloves of garlic, chopped
> ½ small onion, diced

Cook fettuccine according to package directions. Drain and return pasta to pot; add a teaspoon of the olive oil and toss to coat. Meanwhile steam asparagus and drain.

In large skillet over medium-high heat, sauté cherry tomatoes in remaining 2 tablespoons of olive oil until skin begins to crack. Add onion and cook until translucent. Stir in garlic. Thin sauce with pasta liquid to desired consistency. Toss cooked pasta and asparagus into sauce and serve immediately.

<u>Serves 4</u>. About 290 Calories per serving

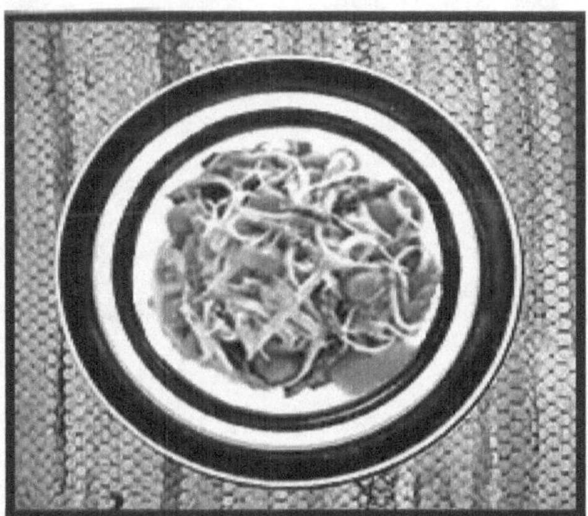

<u>Diet Tip of the Day:</u> A major weight-loss fallacy is that you can **get rid of abdominal fat** by working your abdominal muscles. This is based on the incorrect belief that fat is eliminated from a particular part of your body if you engage the muscles underneath that layer of fat. No such luck.

Barbequed Shrimp & Corn

    1½ pounds large shrimp, peeled and de-veined
    3 Tbsp of your favorite bottled barbeque sauce
    4 medium ears of corn

Pour barbeque sauce into shallow bowl. Toss shrimp in barbeque sauce to coat. Place shrimp on medium-hot grill. Turn shrimp after about two minutes or when shrimp turn pink. Grill until second side turns pink – approximately another 2 minutes. Don't overcook but test a shrimp by cutting to make sure it is cooked through. Salt and pepper to taste. Serve hot or at room temperature.

<u>Serves 4</u>. About 160 Calories per serving (shrimp only).

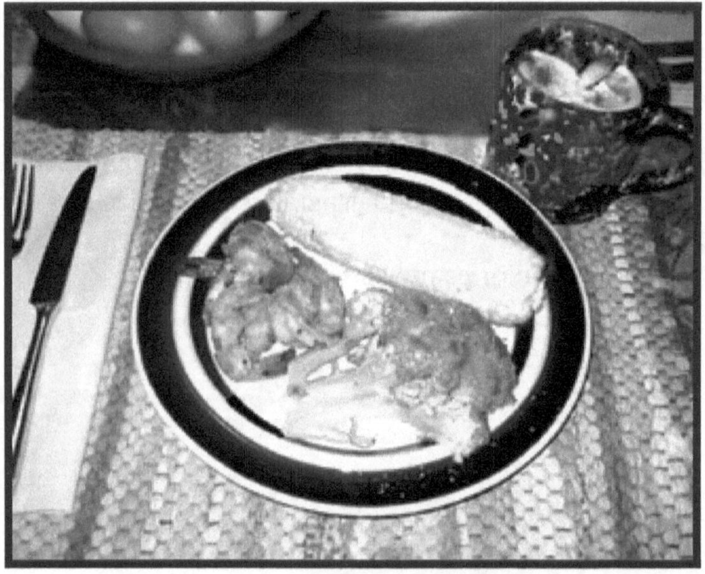

<u>Diet Tip of the Day:</u> A very **important weight-profile parameter** is your waist-to-hip ratio. Health risks for heart attack and stroke increase considerably for men with a ratio above 1.0 and for women with a ratio above 0.8. To calculate your ratio, measure your waist size (at its narrowest circumference) and divide it by your hip size (at the widest section).

Recipe 24

<u>Cheeseburger Heaven</u>

There's really not much to grilling hamburgers. The ideal meat for a juicy burger is ground chuck with about 20% fat, but we are talking diet here. So we opt for leaner, much leaner meat.

1¼ pounds ground sirloin (95% lean)
4 thin slices low-fat American cheese

Mix ground beef in large bowl. Salt and pepper to taste. Divide into 4 equal portions and form burgers about 1-inch thick.

Cook burgers over a hot fire on charcoal or gas-fired grill. For medium, cook about 4 minutes on each side. Top with slice of cheese. Add lettuce and tomato. Season to taste.

<u>Serves 4</u>. About 370 Calories per serving (cheeseburger only).

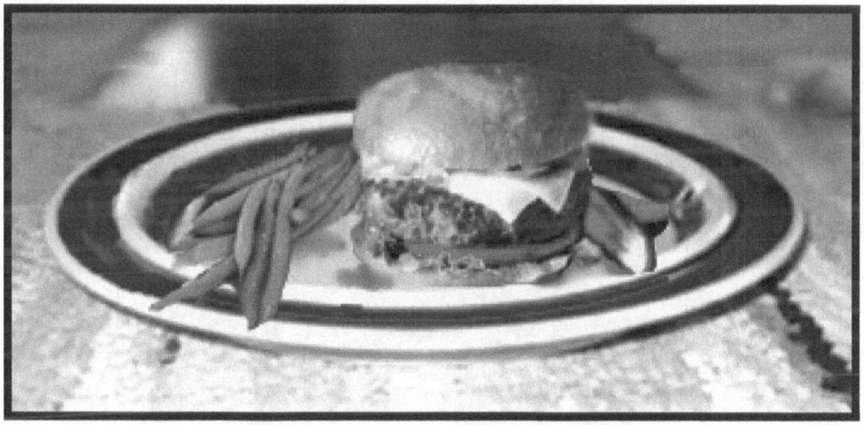

<u>Diet Tip of the Day:</u> **Plan to be on a diet the rest of your life**. Not necessarily a weight reducing diet. At some point you'll want to just maintain your weight. But you will still need to continue to make good healthy food choices – and not slip back to your old eating habits.

Recipe 25

<u>Tina's Baked Sea Bass</u>

    4 4-ounce Chilean sea bass fillets
    ½ pound green beans
    ¾ pint cherry tomatoes (about 20)
    ¾ cup brown rice (prepare per package directions)

<u>Sea Bass:</u> Dust filets with flour. Dip in egg wash & then Panko bread crumbs. Place fillets in baking dish coated with non-stick spray. Bake about 15 minutes in oven preheated to 350 °F.

<u>Green Beans & Tomato:</u> Place green beans in skillet. Add ¼-inch of water and cook over medium heat until water boils off. Add cherry tomatoes and olive oil. Stir well and sauté for a few minutes. Season with fresh rosemary and oregano.

<u>Brown Rice-Pesto mix:</u> Prepare brown rice per package directions. Add 4 teaspoons packaged "green" pesto. Mix thoroughly.

<u>Red Pepper Sauce:</u> Blend one roasted red pepper (skinned), ½ cup non-fat yogurt, 1 tsp lemon juice, 1 Tbsp olive oil, 1 Tbsp chili sauce, and a dash of Worcestershire sauce.

Serves 4. One plate consisting of one sea bass fillet with spooned over red pepper sauce (150 Calories), green beans & tomato mix (75 Calories), brown rice-pesto mix (120 Calories) and half ear of corn (50 Calories) – totals about 395 Calories.

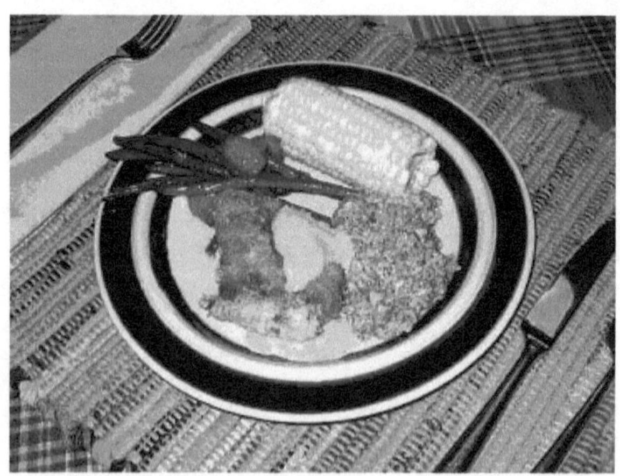

<u>**Diet Tip of the Day:**</u> Protein foods make you **feel full longer** and help prevent overeating.

Recipe 26

<u>Turkey Tenders & Vegetables</u>

    2   turkey breast tenderloins (about 1½ lb)
    1   medium eggplant (about ¾ lb)
    ¾   pound yellow (summer) squash
    2   medium plum tomatoes, quartered

<u>Marinade</u>: Whisk in a bowl 2 tsp lemon zest, ¼ cup lemon juice, 2 Tbsp olive oil, 1 Tbsp chopped garlic, 1 Tbsp chopped rosemary, ¼ tsp salt and a pinch of black pepper. Put marinade and turkey breasts in large re-sealable plastic bag. Refrigerate about 45 minutes

Slice eggplant and squash lengthwise about ½-inch thick. Place with tomatoes on a baking sheet coated with a nonstick spray.

Grill turkey breasts approximately 7 to 9 minutes per side, or until an instant-read thermometer inserted from the side to middle registers 160°F. Slice turkey and set aside.

Grill eggplant and zucchini about 4 minutes per side, or until just tender. Grill tomatoes about 2 minutes per side, or until charred but not soft. Cut vegetables bite-size and toss with remaining marinade. Serve with sliced turkey.

<u>Serves 4</u>. About 350 Calories per serving (includes turkey and veggies)

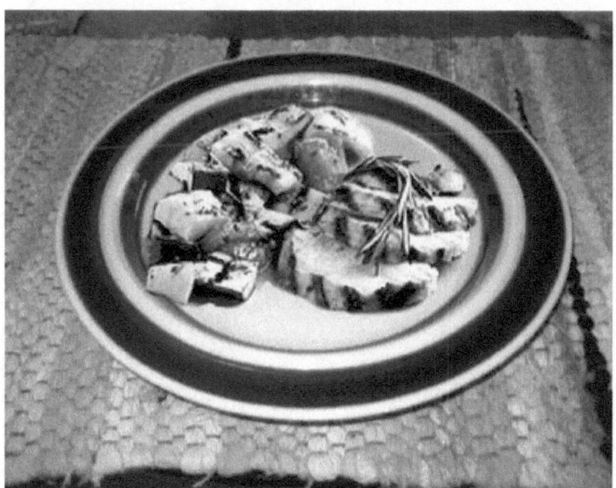

<u>Diet Tip of the Day:</u> It's a lot easier to eat 1,000 Calories than it is to burn 1,000 Calories exercising. So a stroll after dinner probably isn't going to offset the calories you ingested eating a Big Mac plus fries.

Recipe 27

Pasta Rapini

> 2 cloves garlic - coarsely chopped
> 1½ cups of crushed San Marzano tomatoes
> 2 cups Rapini (broccoli rabe)
> 1 tablespoon crushed red pepper flakes (optional)
> ½ pound medium-sized whole grain pasta

Tomato Sauce: In large pan, sauté two tablespoons olive oil over medium-high heat. Add the garlic and sauté until translucent (but not browned). Add crushed San Marzano tomatoes (use plum tomatoes if San Marzano are not available) and bring to a boil. Reduce heat to low and simmer for about 30 minutes or until cooked. Season with salt and pepper. Set aside.

Rapini: Discard the tough stems and slice into 2-inch pieces. Bring a pot of water to a boil. Add Rapini (a variety of the vegetable broccoli rabe) and 1 tablespoon salt. Blanch Rapini about 5 minutes or until slightly cooked but still crunchy at stems. Drain, set aside and cover.

Cook pasta according to package instructions until al dente. Three minutes before pasta is ready, add the Rapini to the sauté pan (containing the tomato sauce). Heat mixture over medium heat. Drain pasta and add it to the pan with the Rapini and tomatoes. Add hot pepper flakes (optional) and toss for 1 to 2 minutes over high heat. Drizzle lightly with extra virgin olive oil and plate. Delicious!

Serves 4. About 290 Calories per serving

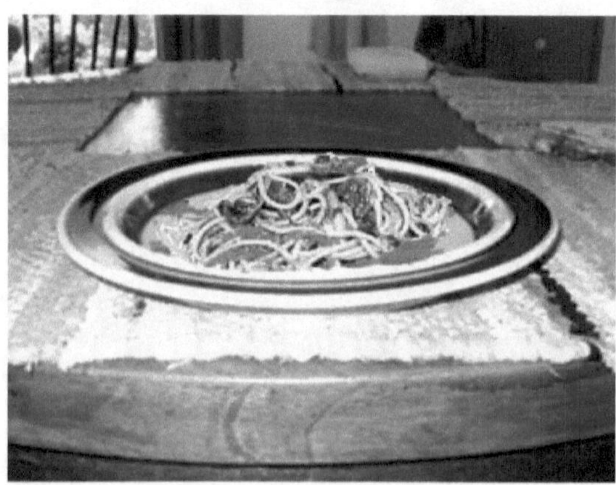

Diet Tip of the Day: Keep a daily food log to **record everything you eat**. For some people it really works wonders.

Recipe 28

Grilled Tilapia

Tilapia is a mild, white fish that inhabits fresh water. This fish has very low levels of mercury because it's fast-growing, short-lived, and mostly eats a vegetarian diet. According to the Monterey Bay Aquarium, choose tilapia farmed in the U.S., in environmentally friendly systems. "Avoid" farmed tilapia from China and Taiwan, where pollution and weak management are a problem.

    4 Tilapia filets (about 6 ounces each)

<u>Marinade</u>: ¾ cup olive oil, ½ lemon, juiced, 1 tablespoons oregano, ½ teaspoon black pepper, ¼ cup red wine vinegar, ½ cup finely chopped parsley, 2 cloves garlic, minced and 2 dashes Tabasco (optional).

Combine all ingredients (except filets) in a large re-sealable plastic bag and shake well. Then place fish filets in the marinade for 30 minutes. Remove fillets from marinade and cook on hot grill for approximately 2 to 3 minutes per side.

<u>Serves 4</u>. About 300 Calories per serving (fish only)

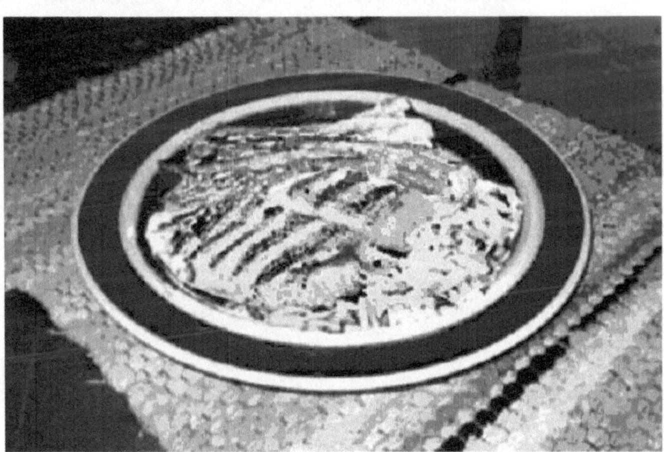

Photo shows two fish filets. Actual serving size is <u>one filet</u>.

<u>Diet Tip of the Day:</u> One serving of asparagus can provide you with 66% of your daily folate needs. Folate is a B-vitamin which is involved with cellular division, and therefore aids the development of a baby's nervous system.

<u>Lo-Cal Beef Stew</u>

    ½ lb beef stew meat, fat trimmed & cut in 1" cubes
    2 celery stalks diced
    1 medium onion diced
    3 large carrots cut into large chunks
    3 large boiling potatoes, peeled & cut in chunks
    ½ up green beans
    1 container beef stock (low sodium)
    2 tablespoons of flour, and 1 tablespoon of olive oil
    ½ teaspoon dried herbs, and 1 bay leaf

Season meat with ½ teaspoon dried herbs, salt and pepper. In a Dutch oven, add olive oil and heat until warm. Add meat, diced onion and celery and cook over medium heat about 5 minutes. Add enough beef stock to cover meat. Bring to a boil. Reduce heat, add bay leaf, cover and simmer over low heat until meat is fork tender (about 1½ hours). Add potatoes and carrots. Cover and cook until vegetables are tender (about 30 min). Add green beans and cook an additional 10 min. Skim off any fat from the surface.

In a small bowl, add small amount of water to 2 tablespoons of flour – and stir. Pour the flour-water mixture into the stew and stir until a thick gravy forms. Taste and adjust seasoning. Spoon approximately ¼ of the stew in each plate.
<u>Serves 4</u>. About 365 Calories per serving

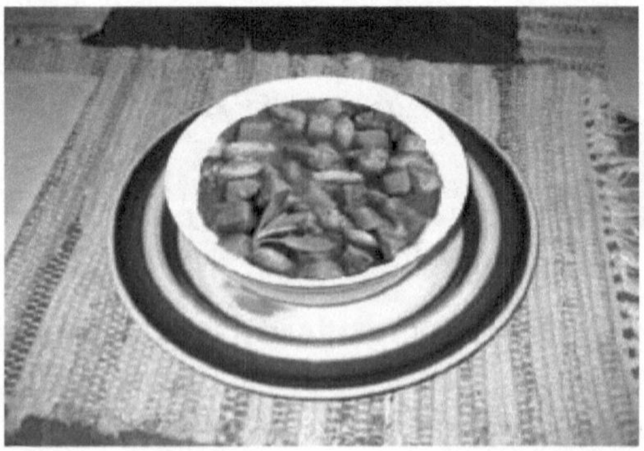

<u>Diet Tip of the Day:</u> **Free-range** animals get more exercise and eat a natural diet, so their meat is usually lower in fat and calories than farm-raised cattle.

Recipe 30

<u>Chicken with Veggies</u>

   4 boneless, skinless chicken breast halves (about 5 oz each)
12 broccoli florets
 1 bunch of asparagus
 2 ripe medium-size tomatoes
 2 tablespoons Lo-Cal (light) salad dressing

Place evenly cut broccoli and asparagus spear in a microwave-safe pan, add a little water to bottom of the pan and top with microwave-safe plastic wrap. (Be sure to pull back one corner of the plastic topper so some steam can escape.) Check veggies periodically and take them out of the microwave when they reach desired softness.

Season chicken breasts evenly with salt and pepper. Heat a large nonstick skillet over medium-high heat. Coat pan with cooking spray. Cook chicken about 4 minutes on each side or until no pink remains.

For each serving, plate one chicken breast and a portion of the steamed broccoli and asparagus. Add one-half of a tomato cut into pieces. Drizzle about 2 tablespoons of a light salad dressing that contains no more than 50 Calories in 2 tablespoons.

<u>Serves 4</u>: One serving of chicken breast halve, veggies & dressing is about 365 Calories.

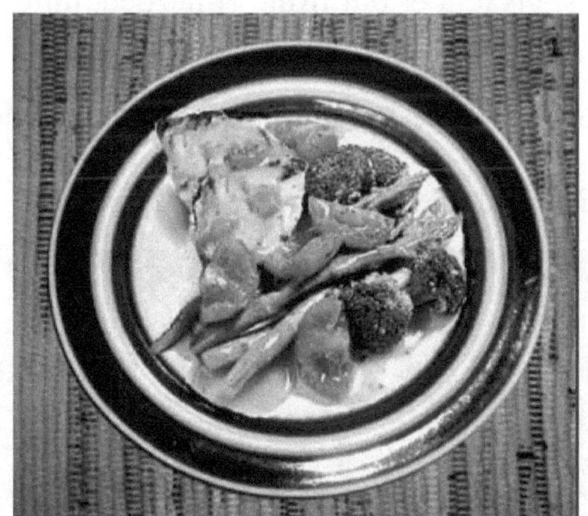

Shown drizzled with Light Thousand Island dressing.

<u>Diet Tip of the Day:</u> Steaming in a microwave oven is one of the best ways to cook veggies so they retain nutrients. Another advantage is the cooking adds no fat or sodium.

Recipe 31

<u>Pasta e Fagioli</u>

This is one variation of a traditional, nutritious peasant dish served all over Italy.

    14.5-oz can whole tomatoes with juice, crushed
14.5-oz can cannellini beans, drained
1 cup of any tube-shaped pasta
2 tablespoon olive oil
1 medium onion, diced
2 cloves garlic, minced
1 stalk celery, finely chopped
3 cups chicken stock
2 cups fresh baby spinach or escarole
1 tsp dried basil
½ teaspoon dried oregano
2 Tbsp fresh parsley, chopped

Heat olive oil, onion and celery in large saucepan over medium heat. Sauté until onions are golden brown. Add garlic and stir constantly for one minute. Pour in tomatoes and their juices and bring to a boil. Add beans and chicken stock and return to a boil. Stir in spinach (or escarole) and seasonings. Simmer for about 5 minutes. Add pasta and cook about 15 minutes or until pasta is tender but firm. If needed, thin soup with hot water.

Ladle into soup bowls. Garnish with grated Parmesan cheese. Salt and pepper to taste.
<u>Serves 4</u>. About 300 Calories per serving.

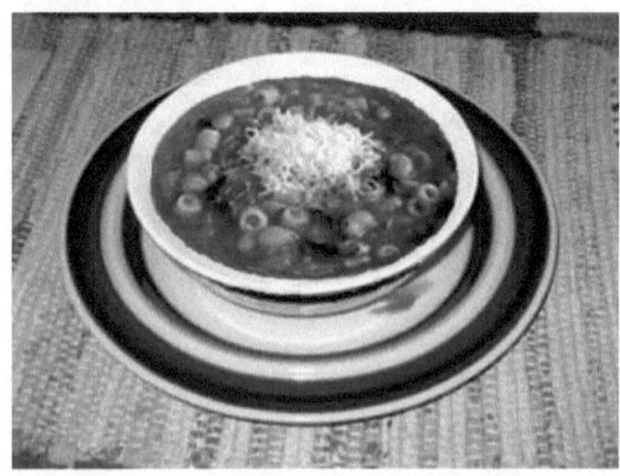

Recipe 32

<u>Beef Kebob</u>

    1 lb boneless beef tenderloin steaks, 1" thick
    8 ounces medium mushrooms
    2 medium bell peppers (any color), cut in pieces
Marinate ingredients:
    2 tablespoons olive oil
    1 tablespoon chopped fresh oregano
    2 cloves garlic, minced
    ½ teaspoon ground black pepper

Cut beef steak into 1-inch square pieces. Combine marinate ingredients in large bowl. Add beef, mushrooms and bell pepper pieces. Toss to coat. Cover bowl and refrigerate for about two hours. Thread beef and vegetable pieces onto eight 12-inch metal skewers.

Grill kebobs over medium-high heat for 8 to 10 minutes, turning occasionally. Check center of meat with a small incision to determine when the meat is done.

Microwave a one-pound package of frozen mixed vegetables. Plate two kebob skewers and about one-quarter of the mixed veggies.

<u>Serves 4</u>. One plate consisting of two kebob skewers (350 Calories) plus ¼ pound of mixed green vegetables (40 Calories) totals about 390 Calories.

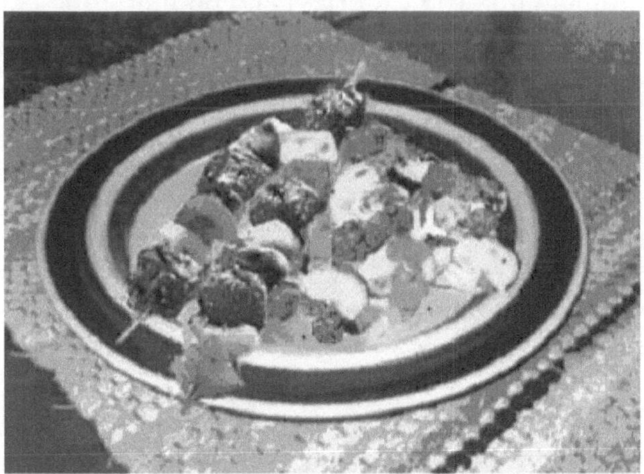

<u>Diet Tip of the Day</u>: Remember your stomach is about the size of your fist. So it doesn't take much food to fill it comfortably.

Recipe 33

Baked Haddock

    4   4-oz haddock fillets (or salmon fillets)
    ½   cup white wine
    ½   cup non-fat yogurt mixed with ¼ cup pureed roasted red pepper
    ½   pound green beans
    ¾   pint cherry tomatoes (about 20)
    1   tablespoon olive oil
    ¾   cup bulgur, prepared per package directions

Lightly dust fillets with flour. Dip in beaten egg white and then in Panko bread crumbs. Brown fillets in non-stick pan. Place fillets skin side down in baking dish coated with non-stick spray. Add white wine and cook in oven preheated to 350 °F for about 15 minutes. Spoon pan juices over fillets. Salt and pepper to taste.

Place green beans in skillet. Add ¼-inch of water and cook over medium heat until water boils off. Add cherry tomatoes and olive oil. Stir well and sauté for a few minutes. Season with fresh rosemary and oregano. Salt and pepper to taste.

Plate haddock fillet and spoon over yogurt-red pepper sauce. Garnish with fresh parsley. Add green beans & tomato mix and the bulgur.   Serve hot.

Serves 4. One plate consisting of one haddock fillet (215 Calories) with green beans & tomato mix (65 Calories) and bulgur (140 Calories) totals 420 Calories.

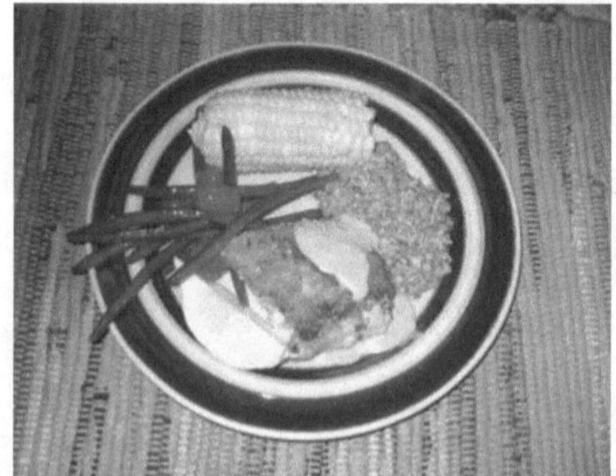

Note that corn-on-the-cob is only for the 1800 Calorie diet.

Diet Tip of the Day: It's much easier to stay with an exercise program when it's done in tandem. So enlist a friend to be your exercise buddy.

<u>Chicken Cacciatore</u>

    ¾ lb skinless, boneless chicken breast halves
    ¼ lb of your favorite pasta
    ½ cup chopped onion
    ½ cup chopped green bell pepper
    14.5-ounce can chopped tomatoes, drained
    8-ounce can tomato sauce
    1½ teaspoons Italian seasoning
    ⅓ cup sliced ripe olives
    ⅛ teaspoon black pepper

Cut chicken breasts into small pieces. Spray a large heavy skillet with olive oil flavored cooking spray.

Sauté chicken, onion and green pepper for 6 to 8 minutes. Stir in drained tomatoes and tomato sauce. Add Italian seasoning, olives and ⅛ teaspoon ground black pepper. Mix well to combine. Lower heat and simmer for 15 to 20 minutes, stirring occasionally.

Cook pasta per package directions. Ladle chicken and sauce over pasta and serve immediately.<u>**Serves 4**</u>. About 310 Calories per serving

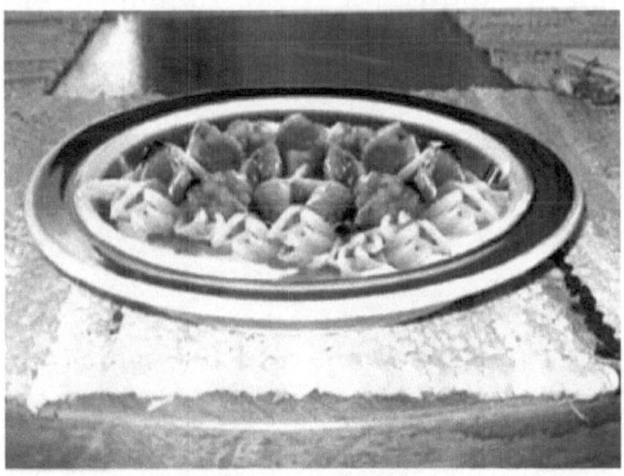

<u>**Diet Tip of the Day**</u>: Inevitably, you're going to be faced with a stressful situation. Instead of turning to food for comfort, be prepared with some non-food tactics that work for you, such as listening to music, reading, writing in a journal, or meditating.

<u>Dawn's Blueberry Muffins</u>

Wholesome whole-grain blueberry muffins just like grandma used to make. Serve them at breakfast, or as a nutritious dessert, or a wonderful snack. (Make a dozen. Have one today and store the remainder in your freezer until they are called for again later in the diet.)

- 4 ounces bran flakes
- ¼ cup sugar
- 1¼ cups whole grain flour
- 1 teaspoon baking soda
- ¼ teaspoon baking powder
- ¼ teaspoon salt
- ½ cup blueberries (fresh or frozen)
- 1 egg, beaten
- 1 cup buttermilk
- ¼ cup vegetable oil

Preheat oven to 400 ºF. Coat muffin tins with nonstick cooking spray. In a bowl combine dry ingredients. In another bowl combine wet ingredients and mix thoroughly. Add wet ingredients to dry ingredients and mix until just blended. Do not over mix. Gently fold in blueberries. Spoon batter into muffin tins until two-thirds full. Bake 15 minutes or until muffin tops are golden brown.

<u>Yield</u> is 12 Muffins, 145 Calories each

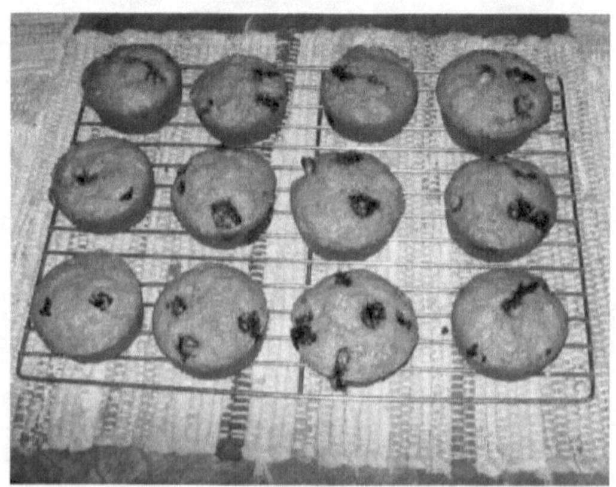

<u>**Diet Tip of the Day:**</u> **Acquire a good low-calorie cookbook**. Be sure the recipes cover breakfast, lunch and dinner, and all the recipes contain nutritional information, especially the calories per serving.

Recipe 35

Poached Cod in Tomato Broth

    2   cups dry white wine
    1   cup clam juice
    2   cans (14.5-ounce) diced tomatoes, drained
    1   small onion, diced
    1   garlic clove, minced
    ½   tsp dried parsley, or sprigs of fresh parsley
    1   bay leaf
    12 black olives, pitted and halved
    4   cod fish fillets (about 6 ounces each)

Note that sole, flounder, halibut or haddock may be substituted for cod.

Use a pan large enough to hold the fish in a single layer. Place all the ingredients except the fish in the pan. Over high heat, bring poaching liquid to a boil (pan uncovered). Reduce heat and simmer the liquid another 6 minutes.

Carefully place the fish filets in the liquid. Cover the pan and reduce heat until liquid is just simmering. Poach until fish are completely opaque and tender – about 8 minutes. Plate fish and ladle broth over fish.
Serves 4. 275 Calories per serving.

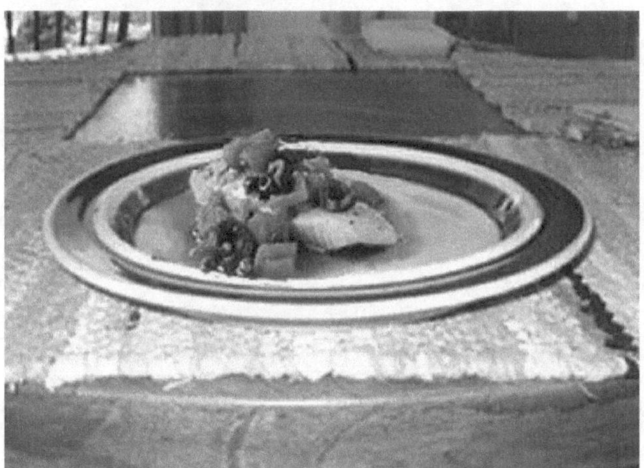

Diet Tip of the Day: A **good reducing diet must help you remain healthy** while you are losing weight.

<u>Chicken Piccata</u>

- 1 pound boneless skinless chicken breast halves
- 2 teaspoons olive oil
- 1 teaspoon minced garlic
- ¼ cup shallots, diced
- ¾ pound fresh green beans, washed and snipped
- 1 teaspoon lemon juice
- ¼ cup capers, rinsed
- 2 fresh lemons, cut into small wedges

In a skillet, heat olive oil and minced garlic over medium heat. Sauté chicken breasts and shallots for two to three minutes, tossing often, until chicken is partially cooked. Add green beans and one teaspoon of lemon juice and sauté for an additional two to three minutes, or until chicken is completely cooked and green beans are al dente. Add capers; and cover chicken. Let sit for one more minute to warm capers. Serve immediately with wedges of lemon.

<u>Serves 4</u>. 270 calories per serving

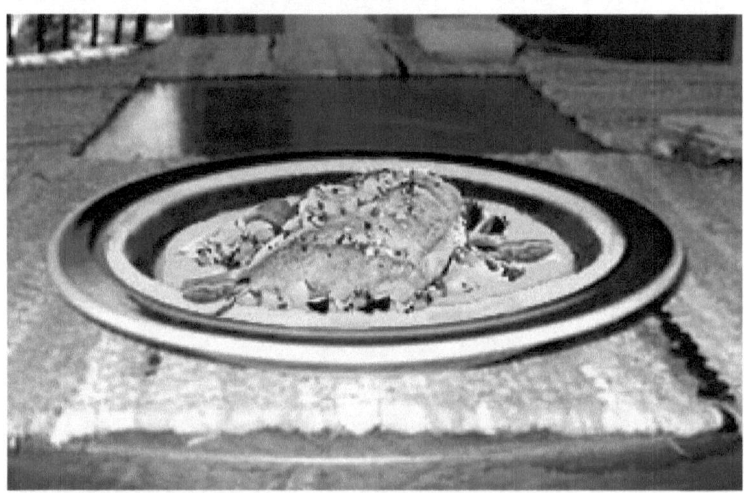

<u>Diet Tip of the Day:</u> Handle **occasional overeating by compensating**. To do this, estimate how far you have strayed from your weight-loss diet and then make amends at the next opportunity (usually the next meal or two) – by eating less.

<h1 style="text-align:center">Recipe 37</h1>

<u>Beans & Greens Salad</u>

⅓ cup chopped oregano
⅓ cup chopped parsley
3 cloves garlic, chopped
1 lemon, juiced

Prepare dressing by combining above ingredients and stirring in ¼ cup extra-virgin olive oil. Salt and pepper to taste.

½ pound mesclun mix
¼ pound green beans
19-ounce can garbanzo beans (chickpeas)

Arrange mesclun mix, garbanzo beans and green beans on a large platter. Drizzle dressing over beans and greens.
<u>Serves 4</u>. Approximately 260 Calories per serving.

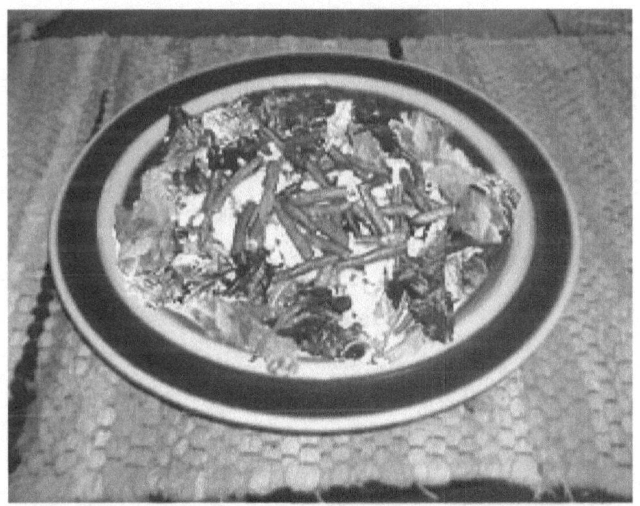

<u>Diet Tip of the Day:</u> **Fat-free isn't always your best bet**. Low fat doesn't always mean low calorie! Most often sugar is substituted for fat and the calorie total remains the same or even higher. Instead, look for low-calorie or reduced-calorie foods.

Recipe 38

Pan-Fried Sole

    4 sole fillets (6-ounces each), skinned
    1 tablespoon olive oil
Salsa Ingredients:
    1 pint cherry tomatoes, quartered
    ¾ cup cucumber, finely chopped
    ⅓ cup yellow bell pepper, finely chopped
    3 tablespoons fresh basil, chopped
    2 tablespoons capers
    1½ tablespoons shallots, finely chopped
    1 tablespoon balsamic vinegar
    2 teaspoons lemon rind, grated
Combine salsa ingredients in a bowl and stir in ½ teaspoon salt and ⅛ teaspoon black pepper. Mix thoroughly.

Heat olive oil in a large nonstick skillet over medium-high heat. Season sole fillets with
½ teaspoon salt and ⅛ teaspoon black pepper. Add fish to pan; cook about 1½ minutes on each side or until fish flakes easily when tested with a fork. Spoon salsa over fish and serve immediately.
Serves 4. 325 Calories per serving

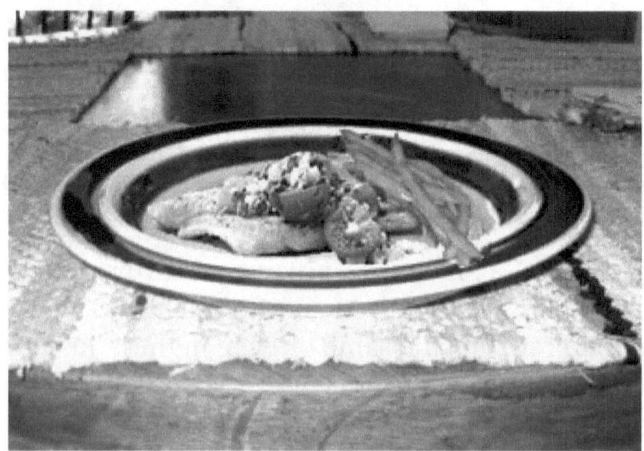

Diet Tip of the Day: If you are overweight start on a weight loss diet now because it will only become **more difficult to lose weight as you get older**.

Beef Steak Strips

 1 lb top loin sirloin, or top round about ¾" thick
 1 tsp garlic, finely chopped
 ½ tsp dry thyme
 ½ tsp salt and ¼ tsp black peppercorns

Cut the steak into 3-inch long by ¼-inch thick strips Sprinkle the beef strips with garlic, thyme, salt and pepper. Prepare a large non-stick skillet over medium-high heat. Add the steak strips and shake the skillet constantly to avoid sticking. Cook approximately 2 to 3 minutes until meat is seared but pink inside. Check the center by making small incision.
Serves 4. About 330 Calories per serving (meat only).

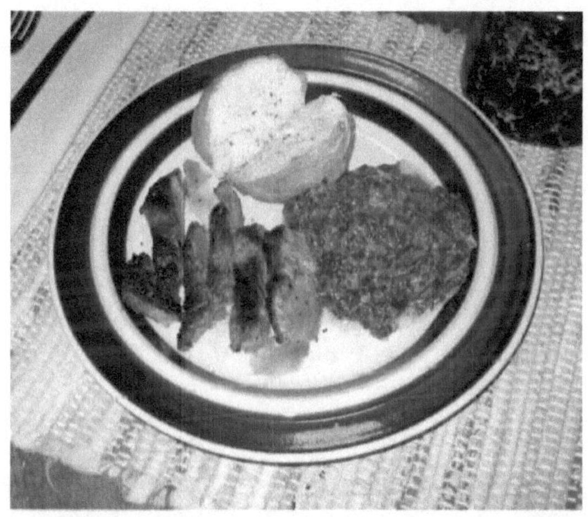

Diet Tip of the Day: Bear in mind, that knowledge and the discipline to **workout regularly** are far more important than fancy equipment.

<u>Grilled Scallops &Polenta</u>

- 1 pound sea scallops
- ¾ cup polenta cornmeal
- ¾ cup skim milk
- 1 medium Portobello mushroom
- ½ pound green beans
- ¼ cup chopped red onion
- 16 asparagus spear
- 1 teaspoon extra-virgin olive oil

Bring 1½ cups of water and skim milk to rapid boil. Add salt to taste and slowly add polenta while stirring. Reduce heat. Continue stirring until desired consistency is reached. Pour polenta into lightly greased pan. After polenta has cooled cover and refrigerate. Cut chilled polenta into 4 pieces. Grill on medium-hot fire – about two minutes on each side.

Brush Portobello mushroom and asparagus spear with olive oil and place on grill for about 3 minutes on each side.

Grill scallops on medium-hot fire. Turn after two minutes or when first side turns opaque. Grill until second side turns opaque – about another 2 minutes. Don't overcook but test a scallop by cutting to make sure it's cooked through. Salt and pepper to taste.

<u>Serves 4</u>. The food on the plate pictured below totals about 380 Calories.

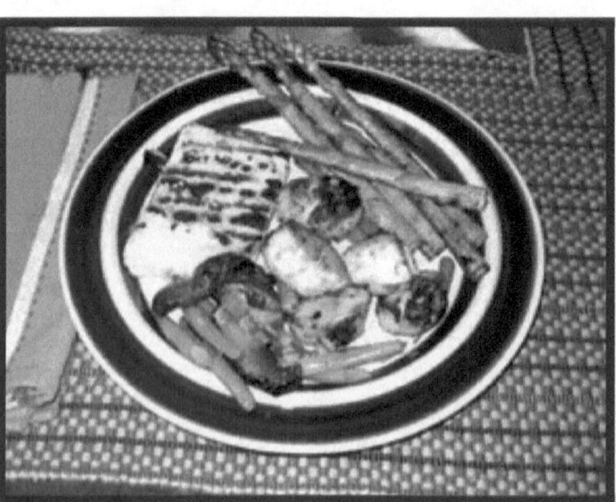

<u>Diet Tip of the Day:</u> Bear in mind, that knowledge and discipline to workout regularly are more important than having access to the fancy equipment in a fitness facility.

<h1 style="text-align:center">Recipe 41</h1>

<u>Pork Chop with Orange Slices</u>

    4   loin pork chops, ½-inch-thick (about 1½ lbs total, including bones)
    8   orange slices, ¼-inch-thick
    1   teaspoon salt
    ¾   teaspoon black pepper
    ¼   cup orange marmalade preserve
    ½   cup bottled fruit-based barbecue sauce
    such as Grandville's Gourmet BBQ Sauce

<u>Marinade</u>: ½ cup orange juice, 2 teaspoons soy sauce and ¼ teaspoon crushed red pepper.

Combine pork chops and marinade in large re-sealable plastic bag. Refrigerate for about 30 minutes. Remove chops from marinade and season with salt and black pepper.

Stir together orange marmalade and BBQ sauce in a small bowl. Brush one side of pork chops evenly with half of marmalade-BBQ mixture. Grill chops, with marmalade-BBQ mixture side up over medium-high heat (about 375°) for about 5 minutes or until done. Turn chops, and brush with remaining marmalade-BBQ mixture. Grill another 5 minutes or until done. Grill orange slices over medium-high heat, 1 minute on each side.
<u>Serves 4</u>. 470 Calories per serving (includes pork chop and two orange slices).

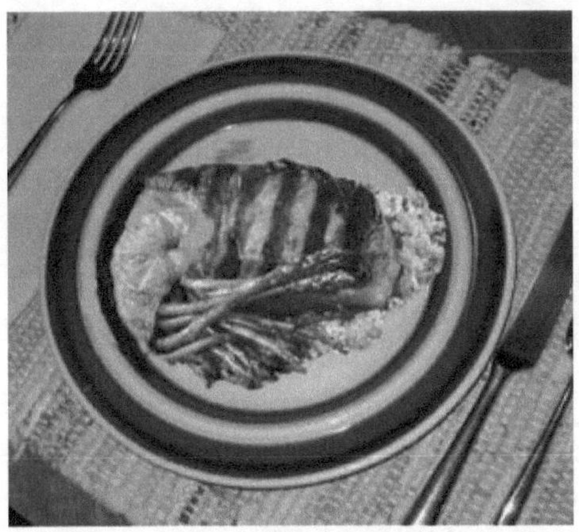

<u>**Diet Tip of the Day:**</u> Make sure fat is trimmed from meat. Most meats are about 80 Calories per ounce – whereas, pure fat is 256 Calories per ounce!

<h1 align="center">Recipe 42a</h1>

<u>Low-Cal Smoothie</u>

Smoothies are delicious, nutritious and fun to drink! They're great for a fast but nutritious breakfast, a light energy-boosting lunch, a healthy snack, a late afternoon pick me up, and a delicious dessert. Making your own smoothie is a smart way to save money and get healthy at the same time!

 8 ounces plain fat-free yogurt
 1 cup orange juice
 1 cup strawberries
 ½ cup blueberries
 1 banana
 1 teaspoon sugar
 1 teaspoon vanilla extract

Place yogurt, strawberries, and blueberries in a blender. Pour in orange juice. Add sugar and vanilla extract to mixture. Blend all ingredients until thick and smooth. Pour smoothie into a glass and enjoy.
<u>Serves 2</u>. About 220 Calories per serving

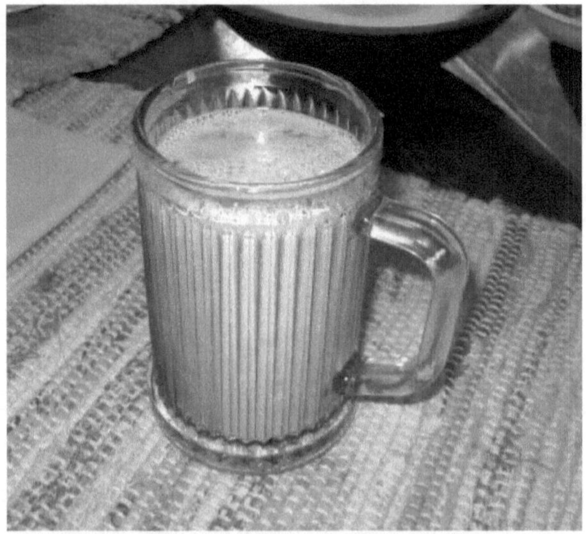

<u>Diet Tip of the Day:</u> Two scientific journals indicate **dark chocolate -** not white chocolate or milk chocolate - is potent antioxidant and is good for you. But don't overdo it, because you have to offset the extra chocolate calories by eating less of other foods.

Recipe 42b

<u>Healthy Pasta Salad</u>

½	pound fusilli pasta, cooked until tender but firm
2	broccoli crowns, chopped
¼	pint cherry tomatoes (about 8), halved
½	cup black olives, halved
½	cup garbanzo beans (chick peas)
½	cup fresh "light" mozzarella, chopped
1	tablespoon basil
1	tablespoon rosemary
2	teaspoons garlic powder
¼	cup of a **recommended dressing** (page 21)

Combine dry ingredients in a medium-size bowl. Stir in salad dressing.
Mix thoroughly. Salt and black pepper to taste.
<u>Serves 4</u>. 370 Calories per serving.

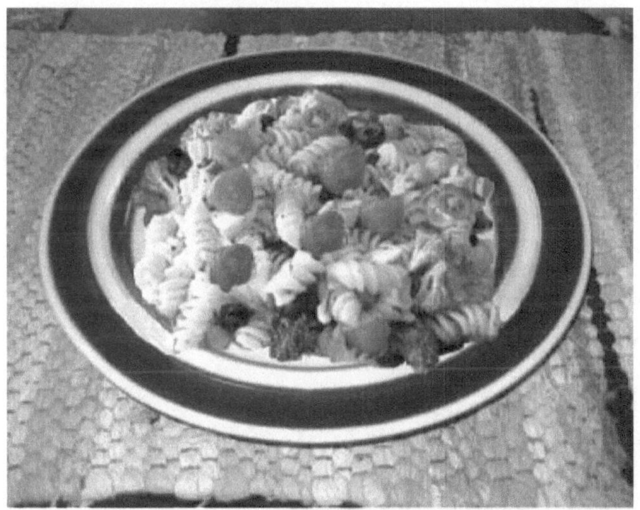

<u>Diet Tip of the Day:</u> Ask yourself: "**Why am I overweight**?"   Do you
eat too much of everything? Too much dessert? Drink too much beer? Is
your only exercise walking from the TV to the refrigerator? Determine the
why and then focus on one or two of your problem areas. Sometimes it's
that simple.

Recipe 43

<u>Beef Burgundy</u>

- 1 lb boneless beef chuck, trimmed & cut in 1" pieces
- 2 large carrots, cut into 1-inch pieces
- 1 medium onion, cut into 1-inch pieces
- 1 tablespoon flour
- 1 tablespoon tomato paste
- 1 clove garlic, crushed
- 1 tablespoon olive oil
- 1 cup dry red wine
- 2 sprigs fresh thyme
- 10 ounces mushrooms, sliced in half
- 8 ounces frozen peas

In Dutch oven, heat oil on medium-high until hot. Add beef and cook 5 to 6 minutes or until beef is browned on all sides. Transfer beef to a bowl. Preheat oven to 325° F. To drippings in Dutch oven, add carrots, garlic, and onion. Stir occasionally and cook 10 minutes or until vegetables are browned and tender. Stir in flour, tomato paste, ½ teaspoon salt, and ¼ teaspoon black pepper, and cook another minute. Add wine and heat to boiling, stirring until browned bits are loosened from bottom of Dutch oven. Return meat and any juices in the bowl to Dutch oven. Add thyme and mushrooms; bring to a boil. Cover and bake 1½ hours or until meat is fork-tender. Discard thyme sprigs. Before stew is done, cook peas per package instructions and add peas to Dutch oven.

<u>Serves 4</u>. 350 Calories per serving

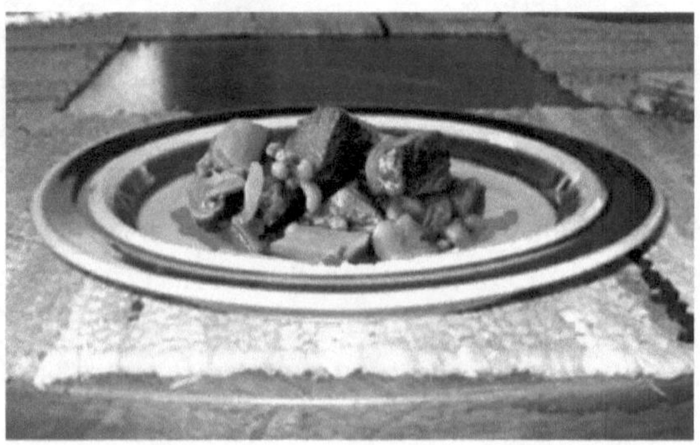

<u>Diet Tip of the Day:</u> When on a diet **simple is better**. Why? Because simple, uncomplicated meals usually contain fewer "hidden calories" than more elaborate dishes.

Recipe 44

<u>Chicken Cutlet</u>

Buy 4 skinless, boneless chicken cutlets or breast halves (about 1 lb), flattened to about ¼ to ½-inch thick.

- ¾ cup Panko bread crumbs
- ⅓ cup grated Parmesan cheese
- 1 egg, beaten
- 4 tablespoons extra-virgin olive oil, divided

Season chicken cutlets with salt and pepper. Combine bread crumbs and Parmesan cheese in a shallow bowl. Whisk egg in a separate shallow bowl. Dip chicken in egg and then coat both sides in crumb mixture.

Heat 2 tablespoons of olive oil in large skillet over medium-high heat. Add 2 cutlets, and cook 2 minutes on each side or until cooked through. Repeat with 2 tablespoons olive oil and remaining 2 cutlets. Serve hot. <u>**Serves 4.**</u> 450 Calories per serving (chicken cutlet only)

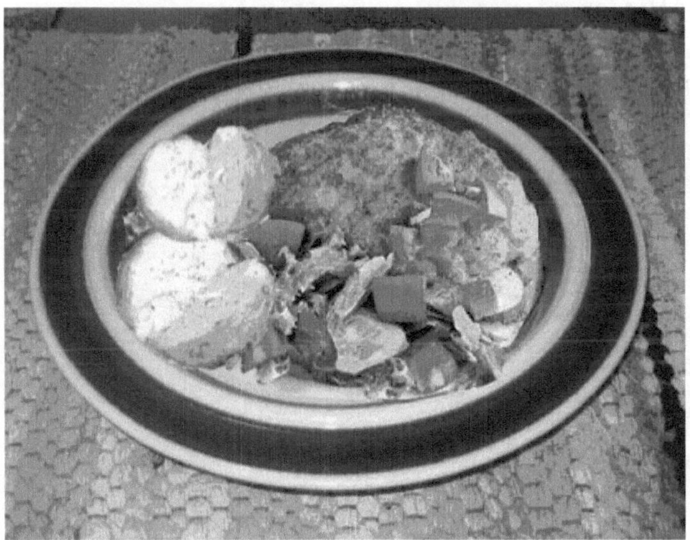

<u>**Diet Tip of the Day:**</u> **Working out at home** has some significant advantages. Your workout takes less time because you don't have to drive back and forth to a fitness facility; and you have the flexibility of dividing your workout into small time segments to fit your day, and working out at home is less expensive.

167

Recipe 45

Personal-Size Meat Loaf

- 1   pound extra lean ground beef
- ⅓ cup quick oats
- 2   egg whites
- ½ cup chipotle salsa, divided
- ¼ cup ketchup, divided

Place egg whites in a large bowl, mixing well with a whisk. Stir in oats, 6 tablespoons salsa, and 2 tablespoons ketchup. Add beef and mix well. Divide beef mixture into 4 equal portions, shaping each into an oval-shaped loaf. and place loaves on baking pan lined with tin foil and coated with cooking spray. Bake in preheated oven at 350°F for 30 minutes or until done.

Combine remaining 2 tablespoons salsa and 2 tablespoons ketchup in a small bowl. Spread mixture evenly over individual meat loaves.
Serves 4. 410 Calories per serving (meat loaf only)

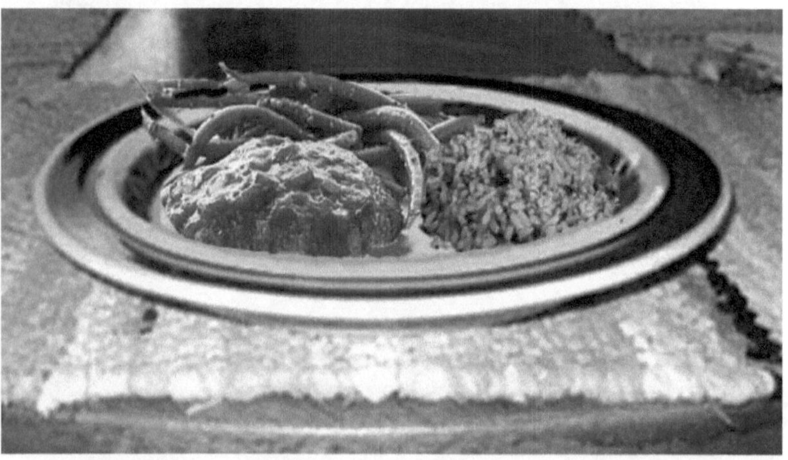

Diet Tip of the Day: To make sure you stay on track, **weigh in once a week**. There may be times when you might not see a weight loss, often because lost fat is temporarily replaced by water. This condition will gradually be corrected as you continue dieting.

Appendix A
Shopping Tips

You will probably have to shop once a week. The following should help you prepare your shopping list.

First, understand that the problem with basing a meal plan on name-brand food items, such as a particular Lean Cuisine frozen entree, is that the item might not be available where you shop, or it may have been discontinued. What to do? That's where Appendices B and D in this book come in handy. Appendix B lists 19 name-brand soups in microwaveable bowls. Appendix D lists more than 140 name-brand frozen meals with their calorie count. Using these lists you should be able to find a substitute for the soup or frozen entree you can't find - a substitute that is based on the same food type, e.g., chicken, fish, or meat, and has the same approximate calorie count.

Substituting Foods

If there is a food listed in the diet you don't like, or perhaps that you forgot to pick up while shopping, you probably can exchange or substitute another food in its place – a technique used by dieticians. Exchanging a food listed in a diet for another food with approximately equal caloric value and nutritional content is the foundation of a successful long-term diet.

Substitution possibilities are almost endless but have to be done carefully. The easiest substitutions are those within the same food group, such as exchanging one vegetable variety for another, or a glass of milk for a cup of yogurt. More sophisticated exchanges cross food groups, for instance replacing 3½ ounces of turkey with a tablespoon of peanut butter spread on a piece of whole wheat bread. Both foods are complete proteins and both contain about 175 Calories. Refer to a good online calorie table to find calorie values. With some understanding and experience, you will be able to substitute foods called for in this diet with equal calorie foods from the same food group.

If there is a food listed in *Maximum Weight Loss* that you don't like, or perhaps that you forgot to pick up while shopping, you probably can exchange or substitute another food in its place – a technique used by dieticians. Exchanging a food listed in a diet for another food with approximately equal caloric value and nutritional content is the foundation of many successful long-term diets. Substitution possibilities are almost endless but have to be done carefully. The easiest substitutions are those within the same food group, such as exchanging one vegetable variety for another, or a glass of milk for a cup of yogurt. More sophisticated exchanges cross food groups, such as replacing 3½ ounces of turkey with a tablespoon of peanut butter on a piece of whole-grain bread. Both foods are complete protein and both contain about 175 Calories. With some understanding and experience, you can use this table to help you substitute foods called for in the *Maximum Weight Loss* with equal calorie foods from the same food group.

Breakfast: You may substitute any cereal for any other wholesome cereal. For example, if you're not crazy about having Shredded Wheat for breakfast on Day 6, substitute Wheat Chex or Cheerios, etc. But remember to adjust the amount of cereal to account for the calorie difference between brands. If you don't like the soft-boiled egg called for on Day 9, cook a fried egg instead. And if Cantaloupe is on the menu but is not in season, replace cantaloupe with a half cup of orange juice – both contain about 50 Calories.

Snacks: Again, where yogurt is specified you may substitute an 6-ounce glass of skim milk, but to maintain a nutritionally balanced diet keep this snack a dairy selection. Similarly, when fruit is on the agenda, you may select any type of fruit but do not stray from the fruit group. Nuts and popcorn can be interchanged at will. Specified convenient brand-name snacks, such as Skinny Cow ice cream, Kashi Granola bars, Nabisco 100 Calorie Pack cookies and Orville Redenbacher's Smart Pop Popcorn should be widely available but other equivalent brands may be substituted if need be. Just make sure the substitute snack has a calorie count that is the same, or very close, to the specified snack.

Another alternative is the following Food Substitution List that suggests substitutions for a variety of food items that appear in the daily meal plans. For example, Day 5 of the diet calls for half a cantaloupe for breakfast. But suppose cantaloupe is not in season, or just doesn't look good, or maybe it's too expensive, or you can't find it at your grocery, from the Food Substitution List you find that you may exchange a ½ cup of orange juice for half cantaloupe – both are in the fruit category and both contain about 50 Calories.

Light Syrup - Use any light syrup (25 Calories per Tbsp)
Big-Bowl Salad - Exchange with unlimited steamed greens (spinach, etc)
Cantaloupe (½) - Use ½ cup Orange juice
Cereal - Exchange with any other whole-grain cereal
Cottage Cheese (1 cup) - Two 8 oz glasses skim milk
Yogurt - Select 6 ounces skim milk
Eggs – Use Egg Beaters

Fresh fruit - ¾ cup canned fruit (no sugar added)
Frozen entrée - Substitute frozen entrée with same calories.
Grapefruit (½) - Choose an orange (medium)
Handful of Nuts - Popcorn Mini Bag
Kashi Chewy Granola Bar - Quaker Chewy Dipps Granola Bar
Kashi Go Lean Waffles - Eggo Nutri-Grain Whole Wheat Frozen Waffles
Hot Pockets Wraps - Lean Pockets Wraps
Morningstar Breakfast Sausage - Any breakfast sausage with
comparable calories
String Cheese - Laughing Cow light cheese (2 wedges)
Popcorn - Use handful of mixed nuts
Raisin bread - Plain whole-grain bread
Skinny Cow Ice Cream Sandwich - Skinny Cow Fudge Ice Cream Bar
Soup - Choose any soup with same calorie count
Whole-grain Bread - Vary bread type (whole wheat, rye, etc)
Wine (4 oz) - Instead select grapes (1 cup)

Shopping Tip: The danger of basing a meal plan on name brand food items, such as frozen entrees, is that the item may not be available where you shop, or it may have been discontinued. What to do? That's where Appendices B, and D, in this book come in handy. **Appendix B** lists 19 name-brand soups in microwaveable bowls. **Appendix D** lists nearly 150 name-brand frozen entrees. Using these lists you should be able to find a substitute for the food you can't find, a substitute that is based on the same food type, e.g., chicken, fish, or meat, and has the same approximate calorie count. So, **if you cannot find the exact item called for in the diet (because it's out of stock or discontinued), substitute a comparable food (of the same type with about the same caloric value).**

In summary, remember that whenever you encounter a product on this diet, such as "Skinny Cow Ice Cream Sandwich" or "Kashi Go Lean Waffles," that has been discontinued or is out of stock, substitute an equivalent food or desert that is of approximately equal caloric value and nutritional content. In other words substitute a different ice cream product for the "Skinny Cow Ice Cream Sandwich" or a another waffle brand for the "Kashi Go Lean Waffles."

Appendix B
Soup SElections

When the Daily Meal Plan menu specifies soup have only one serving (8 ounces) unless stated otherwise. Note that the listed soups were available in most supermarkets as of 09/24/2020.   *These are a canned soup selections.

Soup Description	Calories
Healthy Choice Chicken with Rice	90
Campbell's Tomato	100
Healthy Choice Country Vegetable	100
Progresso Minestrone*	110
Progresso Chickarina*	110
Progresso Italian-Style Wedding*	120
Campbell's Home-Style Light Chicken Corn Chowder*	120
Campbell's Home-Style Chicken Noodle	130
Campbell's Home-Style Butter Nut Squash*	130
Campbell's Healthy Request Vegetable Beef	140
Progresso Lentil*	140
Progresso Green Split Pea*	150
Campbell's Slow Kettle New England Clam Chowder	160
Progresso Macaroni and Bean*	160
Progresso New England Clam Chowder*	170
Progresso Lasagna-Style*	170
Progresso Broccoli Cheese with Bacon*	180
As an alternative, have 2 servings of a 90 Cal soup	180
Campbell's Chunky Classic Chicken Noodle	190
Amy's Rustic Italian Vegetable*	190
Campbell's Chunky Beef n Cheese*	200
Amy's French Country Vegetable*	210
Campbell's Chunky Sirloin Burger + Vegetables	220
Enjoy two servings of a 110 or 120 Calorie soup	230
Enjoy two servings of a 120 Calorie soup	240

Appendix C
Important Frozen
Food Information

Busy families, singles, older people, and office workers alike enjoy the simplicity and convenience of a frozen meal. Many offices have an employee freezer jammed with all kinds frozen meals, which get zapped in a microwave for a quick, portable, portion-controlled, and relatively inexpensive lunch.

In some cases, frozen may actually be better than fresh, because if you keep fresh fruit and vegetables your fridge for a long time, they lose some of their nutritional value. Whereas, frozen foods are usually processed and packaged within hours of being picked. And the freezing process itself does not destroy nutrients. So buying frozen and then defrosting when you want the fruit or vegetable can actually retain more nutrients.

Storing Frozen Foods

According to the U.S. Department of Agriculture, food stored continuously at 0°F is always safe to eat. Freezing keeps food safe and preserves food for extended periods because it prevents the growth of microorganisms that cause both food spoilage and food-borne illness.

Use an appliance thermometer to monitor your freezer's temperature. If a refrigerator freezing compartment can't maintain 0 °F or if the freezer door is opened frequently, use it for short-term food storage, and eat those foods as soon as possible for best quality. Use a free-standing freezer set at 0 °F or below for long-term storage of frozen foods. Again, keep a thermometer in your freezing compartment or freezer to check the temperature.

Because freezing keeps food safe almost indefinitely, recommended freezer storage times are to preserve quality (taste, etc) of food, not the safety or nutritional value. **The quality of frozen dinners or entrees in a freezer at 0 °F will be maintained for 3 to 4 months**.

If there is a power outage, or if your freezer fails, or if the freezer door is left ajar by mistake, the food may still be safe to use. As long as a freezer with its door ajar continues to run, to cool, the foods should stay safe overnight. If a repairman is on the way or it appears the power will be restored soon, just keep your freezer door closed. A freezer full of food will usually keep about 2 days if the door is kept shut; a half-full freezer will last about a day. The freezing compartment of a refrigerator may not keep foods frozen as long. If the freezer is not full, group packages together to help maintain their low temperature.

During a power failure, you may want to put dry ice, a block or bags of ice in the freezer, or transfer foods to a friend's freezer until power returns. Again, use an appliance thermometer to monitor the temperature. To determine the safety of foods when the power goes on, check their condition and temperature. If food is partly frozen, still has ice crystals, or is as cold as if it were in a refrigerator (40 °F), it is safe to refreeze or use. It's not necessary to cook raw foods before refreezing. **If in doubt discard the food. And always discard frozen food whose temperature has exceeded 40 °F for more than two hours.**

Frozen Food Safety

Increasingly, food giants like ConAgra, Nestlé and others that supply Americans with processed foods concede that they cannot ensure the safety of their food products. Frozen foods pose a particularly serious safety problem because unsuspecting consumers buy frozen foods for their convenience and incorrectly believe that cooking frozen foods is a matter of taste – not safety.

Still the food industry says that extensive outbreaks of food-borne illness are rare, even though it is well-known that most of the millions of cases of food-borne illness every year go unreported or are not traced to the source. For example, each year approximately 40,000 cases of salmonella poisoning are reported in the United States – but perhaps as many as one million cases go unreported. (Salmonella is a type of bacteria most often found in poultry, eggs, unprocessed milk, meat and water.) Recently salmonella pathogens in some frozen meals have sickened thousands of people.

How could this happen? First, the supply chain for ingredients in processed foods – from flour to fruits and vegetables to flavorings – is becoming more complex and global in the drive to keep food costs down. As a result, government and industry officials concede that almost every food ingredient is now a potential carrier of pathogens. A further complication is that a large number of food companies subcontract processing work to save money and don't require suppliers to test for pathogens. In fact, companies often don't even know who is supplying their ingredients.

In addition, many frozen-food manufacturers have stopped cooking their products at high temperatures, a tactic they call the "kill step," which is intended to eliminate any lingering microbes. Frequently this process step turns some of the frozen food ingredients into mush. So, instead the "kill step" has been shifted to consumers. For example, ConAgra has added food safety instructions to its frozen meals, including the Healthy Choice brand. A typical "frozen-food safety" instruction offers this guidance: "Internal temperature needs to reach 165°F as measured by a food thermometer in several spots." Moreover, General Mills, now advises consumers to avoid microwaves altogether and cook their frozen pizzas only in a conventional oven. **Bottom line**: To be safe, always cook frozen foods so that the internal temperature reaches 165°F as measured by a good food thermometer.

The Sodium Problem

Sodium and sodium chloride (salt) normally occur in small quantities in many natural foods. People also add salt during food preparation and to the food they eat. But the average sodium intake for American adults is about 3,400 mg daily – more than 1,000 mg higher than the upper limit of 2,400 mg per day recommended by the U.S. Department of Health and Human Services and the Department of Agriculture Dietary Guidelines. (Note that one level teaspoon of salt contains about 2,300 mg of sodium.)

Although sodium plays an important role in your body, many studies have demonstrated that high sodium intake results in excessive water retention which causes blood volume to expand which in turn raises blood pressure. Moreover, some people are more sensitive to the effects of sodium than are others. These sodium-sensitive people retain sodium more easily. If you're in that group, extra sodium in your diet increases your chance of developing high blood pressure, a condition that can lead to cardiovascular and kidney diseases. Individuals who have high blood pressure and who are also salt sensitive are frequently advised to limit their sodium intake even further.

The downside to commercially prepared frozen entrees is that they frequently are loaded with too much salt (sodium). Be aware that, because of the relatively high sodium content of the frozen dinners and microwaveable soups, *Maximum Weight Loss* **diet may not be appropriate for everyone.** When you have your pre-diet medical checkup let your physician know that the <u>no-cooking section</u> of *Maximum Weight Loss* relies to a large degree on commercially processed convenience foods (frozen and microwaveable) – some of which have a relatively high salt (sodium) content.

Appendix D
Frozen Entrees

Appendix D lists three popular brands of frozen entrées: Healthy Choice, Lean Cuisine and Smart Ones. The listing is further divided by entrée type: Poultry, Meat, Seafood, Pasta, Pizza and Other entrées. The entire table is arranged from the lowest to highest in calories. Note that the listed frozen entrées were available in most super markets as of 02/14/2020.

Entrée Type	Name	Brand	Calories
Poultry	Tomato Basil Chicken & Spinach	Smart Ones	160
Meat	Steak Portobella	Lean Cuisine	160
Meat	Asian Style Beef & Broccoli	Smart Ones	~~160~~ 170
Poultry	Herb Roasted Chicken	Lean Cuisine	170
Poultry	Slow Roasted Turkey Breast	Smart Ones	170
Poultry	Grilled Chicken Marsala	Healthy Choice	180
Poultry	Creamy Basil Chicken w Broccoli	Smart Ones	~~180~~ 170
Poultry	Garlic Chicken Rolls	Lean Cuisine	180
Meat	Beef Merlot	Healthy Choice	180
Meat	Homestyle Beef Pot Roast	Smart Ones	180
Poultry	Roasted Turkey & Vegetables	Lean Cuisine	190
Poultry	Chicken & Broccoli Alfredo	Healthy Choice	190
Poultry	Chicken & Vegetable Stir Fry	Healthy Choice	190
Other	Broccoli & Cheddar Roast Potato	Smart Ones	190
Poultry	Home Style Chicken & Potatoes	Healthy Choice	200
Poultry	Crustless Chicken Pot Pie	Smart Ones	~~200~~ 190
Poultry	Buffalo Style Chicken	Lean Cuisine	~~200~~ 190
Pasta	Angel Hair Marinara	Smart Ones	200
Poultry	Salisbury Steak	Smart Ones	200
Meat	Roast Beef & Mashed Potatoes	Smart Ones	~~220~~ 200
Pasta	Primavera Pasta	Smart Ones	210
Poultry	Honey Balsamic Chicken	Healthy Choice	210

Entrée Type	Name	Brand	Calories
Pasta	Ravioli Florentine	Smart Ones	210
Poultry	Cajun Style Chicken & Shrimp	Healthy Choice	220
Pasta	Cheese Ravioli Mushroom Sauce	Smart Ones	230
Poultry	Ranchero Chicken Wrap	Smart Ones	230
Poultry	Lemon Herb Chicken Picante	Smart Ones	230
Pasta	Cheese Ravioli Mushroom Sauce	Smart Ones	230
Meat	Meat Loaf with Mashed Potatoes	Lean Cuisine	~~230~~ 240
Seafood	Shrimp Alfredo	Lean Cuisine	~~230~~ 240
Poultry	Chicken Margherita	Smart Ones	~~220~~ 240
Poultry	Grilled Chicken Caesar	Lean Cuisine	240
Poultry	Honey Glazed Turkey & Potatoes	Healthy Choice	240
Pasta	Spicy Penne Arrabbiata	Lean Cuisine	240
Pasta	Four Cheese Cannelloni	Lean Cuisine	~~240~~ 250
Poultry	Creamy Basil Chicken w Tortellini	Lean Cuisine	~~240~~ 250
Pasta	Cheese Ravioli	Lean Cuisine	250
Pasta	Vermont Cheddar Mac & Cheese	Lean Cuisine	250
Pasta	Fettuccini Alfredo	Smart Ones	250
Poultry	Oriental Chicken	Smart Ones	250
Poultry	Fiesta Grilled Chicken	Lean Cuisine	250
Pasta	Chicken Linguini Red Pepper	Healthy Choice	250
Poultry	Golden Roasted Turkey Breast	Healthy Choice	250
Poultry	Chicken Mesquite	Smart Ones	250
Poultry	Chicken Oriental	Smart Ones	250
Poultry	Orange Sesame Chicken	Smart Ones	250
Poultry	Baked Chicken	Lean Cuisine	~~250~~ 260
Poultry	Teriyaki Chicken & Vegetables	Smart Ones	~~250~~ 260
Seafood	Tuna Noodle Casserole	Smart Ones	~~250~~ 270
Pasta	Spaghetti with Meatballs	Lean Cuisine	260

Entrée Type	Name	Brand	Calories
Poultry	Creamy Chicken & Noodles	Healthy Choice	260
Meat	Barbecue Steak w Red Potatoes	Healthy Choice	260
Pasta	Tortellini Primavera Parmesan	Healthy Choice	260
Pasta	Sesame Noodles with Vegetables	Smart Ones	~~260~~ 280
Pasta	Creamy Rigatoni w Chicken	Smart Ones	260
Pasta	Macaroni & Cheese	Smart Ones	260
Pasta	Butternut Squash Ravioli	Lean Cuisine	260
Other	Santa Fe Rice & Beans	Smart Ones	260
Other	Coconut Chickpea Curry	Lean Cuisine	260
Poultry	Glazed Turkey Tenderloins	Lean Cuisine	270
Poultry	Kung Pao Chicken	Healthy Choice	270
Poultry	Chicken Margherita w Balsamic	Healthy Choice	270
Poultry	Chicken Strips & Sweet Potatoes	Smart Ones	270
Pasta	Spaghetti with Meat Sauce	Smart Ones	~~270~~ 280
Meat	Salisbury Steak with Mac & Cheese	Lean Cuisine	~~270~~ 290
Pasta	Penne Rosa	Lean Cuisine	270
Poultry	Turkey Breast & Stuffing	Smart Ones	~~270~~ 280
Pasta	Classic Macaroni & Beef	Lean Cuisine	270
Pasta	Mushroom Mezzaluna Ravioli	Lean Cuisine	270
Pasta	Pasta with Swedish Meatballs	Smart Ones	~~280~~ 290
Other	Asian Pot Stickers	Lean Cuisine	280
Poultry	Sesame Stir Fry with Chicken	Lean Cuisine	280
Poultry	Roasted Turkey Breast	Lean Cuisine	~~280~~ 290
Poultry	Apple Cranberry Chicken	Lean Cuisine	280
Poultry	Chicken Fettuccini Alfredo	Healthy Choice	280
Poultry	Grilled Chicken Marinara	Healthy Choice	280
Poultry	Sweet & Spicy Orange Chicken	Healthy Choice	280
Poultry	Chicken Parmesan	Smart Ones	280
Poultry	Turkey Breast with Stuffing	Smart Ones	280

Entrée Type	Name	Brand	Calories
Meat	Beef & Broccoli	Healthy Choice	280
Meat	Meatball Marinara	Healthy Choice	280
Meat	Beef Teriyaki	Healthy Choice	280
Pasta	Spinach Artichoke Ravioli	Lean Cuisine	280
Other	Vegetable Fried Rice	Smart Ones	280
Pasta	Spinach Artichoke Ravioli	Lean Cuisine	280
Pasta	Linguini with Ricotta & Spinach	Lean Cuisine	280
Poultry	Chicken Fettuccini	Lean Cuisine	~~290~~ 280
Pasta	Spaghetti & Meatballs	Healthy Choice	280
Pasta	Spaghetti with Meat Sauce	Smart Ones	280
Other	Vegetable Fried Rice	Smart Ones	280
Other	Asian Pot Stickers	Lean Cuisine	280
Poultry	Chicken with Almonds	Lean Cuisine	290
Poultry	Chicken with Peanut Sauce	Lean Cuisine	290
Seafood	Shrimp & Angel Hair Pasta	Lean Cuisine	~~280~~ 290
Poultry	Grilled Chicken Pesto w Veggies	Healthy Choice	290
Poultry	General Tso's Spicy Chicken	Healthy Choice	290
Poultry	Pineapple Chicken	Healthy Choice	290
Poultry	Chicken Enchiladas Suiza	Smart Ones	290
Meat	Swedish Meatballs	Lean Cuisine	290
Seafood	Lemon Pepper Fish	Healthy Choice	290
Pasta	Pasta with Swedish Meatballs	Smart Ones	290
Other	Santa Fe Rice & Beans	Smart Ones	290
Pizza	Thin Crust Cheese Pizza	Smart Ones	290
Seafood	Parmesan Crusted Fish	Lean Cuisine	~~290~~ 300
Pasta	Santa Fe-Style Rice & Beans	Lean Cuisine	~~280~~ 300
Poultry	Roasted Turkey & Vegetables	Lean Cuisine	~~290~~ 300
Poultry	Sweet & Sour Chicken	Lean Cuisine	300
Poultry	Crustless Chicken Pot Pie	Healthy Choice	300

Entrée Type	Name	Brand	Calories
Poultry	Sweet Sesame Chicken	Healthy Choice	300
Poultry	Chicken Fettuccini	Smart Ones	300
Poultry	General Tso's Chicken	Smart Ones	300
Meat	Classic Meat Loaf	Healthy Choice	300
Seafood	Tortilla Crusted Fish	Lean Cuisine	~~300~~ 310
Pasta	Tuscan-Style Vegetable Lasagna	Lean Cuisine	~~300~~ 310
Pasta	Tortellini with Red Pepper Sauce	Lean Cuisine	300
Pasta	Broccoli Cheddar Rotini	Lean Cuisine	300
Pasta	Three Cheese Ziti Marinara	Smart Ones	300
Pasta	Lasagna Florentine	Smart Ones	~~310~~ 300
Seafood	Tortilla Crusted Fish	Lean Cuisine	~~300~~ 310
Pasta	Tuscan-Style Vegetable Lasagna	Lean Cuisine	~~300~~ 310
Poultry	Chicken Fried Rice	Lean Cuisine	~~300~~ 310
Poultry	Orange Chicken	Lean Cuisine	310
Poultry	Chicken Tikka Masala	Lean Cuisine	310
Poultry	Chicken Strips & Fries	Smart Ones	310
Poultry	Chicken Teriyaki	Lean Cuisine	310
Pizza	Thin Crust Pepperoni Pizza	Smart Ones	310
Pasta	Three Cheese Macaroni	Smart Ones	310
Pizza	French Bread Pepperoni Pizza	Lean Cuisine	310
Poultry	Chicken Spinach Mushroom Panini	Lean Cuisine	~~350~~ 310
Other	Spicy Beef & Bean Enchilada	Lean Cuisine	310
Poultry	Chicken Fried Rice	Healthy Choice	320
Meat	Sweet & Spicy Korean Beef	Lean Cuisine	320
Pizza	Farmers Market Pizza	Lean Cuisine	320
Pizza	Margherita Pizza	Lean Cuisine	320
Poultry	Chicken Carbonara	Lean Cuisine	330
Poultry	Mango Chicken w Coconut Rice	Lean Cuisine	330
Poultry	Country Fried Chicken	Healthy Choice	330

Entrée Type	Name	Brand	Calories
Other	Cheese & Fire-Roasted Tamale	Lean Cuisine	330
Poultry	Chicken Club Panini	Lean Cuisine	~~350~~ 340
Meat	Philly Style Steak & Cheese Panini	Lean Cuisine	~~330~~ 350
Poultry	Chicken Parmigiana	Healthy Choice	360
Poultry	Chicken Pecan	Lean Cuisine	~~320~~ 370
Poultry	Sweet & Sour Chicken	Healthy Choice	390
Pizza	Supreme Pizza	Lean Cuisine	~~330~~ 390

Disclaimer

This book offers general meal planning, nutrition and weight control information. It is not a medical manual and the author does not claim to be medically qualified. The material in this book is not intended to be a substitute for medical counseling. Everyone should have a medical checkup before beginning a weight loss program. Moreover, the physician conducting the medical exam should be made aware of and should approve the specific weight control program planned. Additionally, while the author and publisher have made every effort to ensure the accuracy of the information in this book, they make no representations or warranties regarding its accuracy or completeness. Further, neither the author nor publisher assume liability for any medical problems that might result from applying the methods in this book, or for any loss of profit, or any other commercial damages, including but not limited to special, incidental, consequential or other damages, and any such liability is hereby expressly disclaimed.

Vincent W. Antonetti, Ph.D. is an emeritus professor at Manhattan College. He is a weight control and fitness expert who has lectured on fitness at IBM

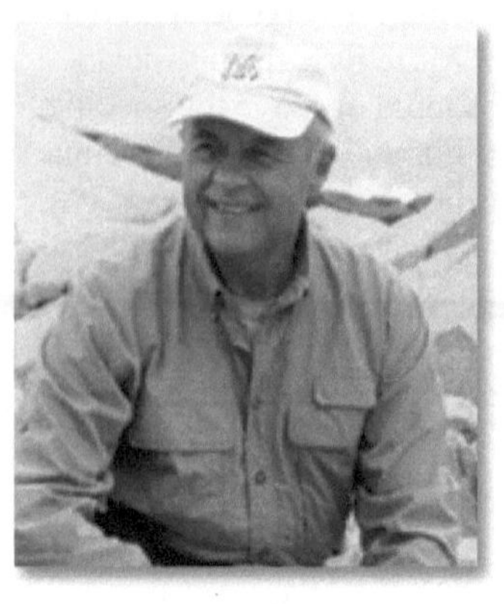

Management and Professional Development classes and often speaks on fitness and weight control. Among his many publications is his highly regarded "The Equations Governing Weight Change in Human Beings," published in the prestigious American Journal of Clinical Nutrition. This paper was the first to develop an accurate equation to calculate weight loss. Dr. Antonetti's critically acclaimed book The Computer Diet was given Consumer Guide magazine's highest recommendation. Recently, Dr. Antonetti coauthored "A Computational Tool to Simulate Energy Balance Components in Pharmacological Interventions," presented at Obesity Week 2016. He also co-authored (with Professor Diana Thomas) "Dynamic Modeling of Energy Expenditure to Estimate Dietary Energy Intake," Chapter 12 in Advances in the Assessment of Dietary Intake, published July 2017 by CRC Press. He is the author or co-author of more than 100 eBooks and paperbacks.

Professor Antonetti is a life long exercise and nutrition enthusiast. Although a senior citizen he still maintains a vigorous physical fitness program - and has managed to maintain his weight to within 2 lbs (about one kg) of the 154 lbs (70 kg) it was when he graduated from college many years ago. He is now semi-retired and living in The Villages, Florida.